FOOD AND BEVERAGE CONSUMPTION AND HEALTH

POMEGRANATES

OLD AGE REMEDY FOR TODAY'S DISEASES

FOOD AND BEVERAGE CONSUMPTION AND HEALTH

Additional books in this series can be found on Nova's website under the Series tab.

Additional e-books in this series can be found on Nova's website under the e-book tab.

FOOD AND BEVERAGE CONSUMPTION AND HEALTH

POMEGRANATES

OLD AGE REMEDY FOR TODAY'S DISEASES

NADY BRAIDY

nova publishers
New York

Additional color graphics may be available in the e-book version of this book.

Library of Congress Cataloging-in-Publication Data

ISBN: 978-1-63463-456-4
Library of Congress Control Number: 2014955185

Published by Nova Science Publishers, Inc. † New York

CONTENTS

PREFACE

Since ancient times, pomegranates have been frequently used as treatments for common ailments in the oldest cultures of the Indus Valley, ancient China, and classical Greece, as well as in the Middle East. The chemical composition and pharmacology of pomegranate constituents is of great interest to life scientists in the modern world. The present book will provide substantial evidence for the beneficial effect of pomegranates on cardiovascular disease by promoting the production of the potent vasodilator, nitric oxide in endothelial cells. It also discusses the neuroprotective effects of pomegranates in brain cells relevant for the management of neurodegenerative disorders such as Alzheimer's disease, Parkinson's disease, and Amyotropic Lateral Sclerosis. It also emphasizes the anti-proliferative and pro-apoptotic properties of pomegranates that are useful for the treatment of several cancers, including malignant tumors of the brain both in vitro and in vivo. Owing to the health benefits of pomegranates, the author also includes a chapter on the cultivation and production of pomegranates

Chapter 1

POMEGRANATES AS A MEDICINAL FRUIT

ABSTRACT

The pomegranate has been deeply associated with the cultures of the Mediterranean region and Near East, where it is savoured as a delicacy and is an important dietary component, revered in symbolism, and greatly appreciated for its medicinal properties. It is strange that a horticultural icon of such importance has been largely relegated to an ornamental role in the United States and much of Europe. Recent trends indicate that the health-giving and flavour filled properties of these fruits may soon reverse this oversight.

INTRODUCTION

Pomegranates belong to the subclass Rosidae, order Myrtales, which is home to a few other fruits such as the guava (Psidium sp.) and feijoa (Feijoa sp.). However, pomegranate is unusual in being one of only two species in its genus, Punica, which is the sole genus in the family Punicaceae (ITIS, 2006). Recent molecular studies suggest a taxonomic reconsideration might place Punica within the Lythraceae [1]. The second species in Punica, P. protopunica, is found only on the island of Socotra, of theArabian Peninsula, and is considered an ancestral species [2] or an independent evolutionary path [3].

The name Punica is the feminized Roman name for Carthage, the ancient city in northern Tunisia from which the best pomegranates came to Italy. It was initially known as Malum punicum, the apple of Carthage. But Linneaus selected the current name, with the specific epithet granatum, meaning seedy or grainy. Its common name in the United States, therefore, means "seedy apple" [4]. While considering naming, it is interesting to note that the fruit's name in French, "grenade", provided the name for the weapon because of similarities in appearance [4].

History of Cultivation

The pomegranate is widely considered native in the region from Iran to northern India with apparently wild plants in many forests of these areas. Others suggest that it is native to the smaller area of Iran and vicinity, and were spread by human movement to a much broader area in prehistory [4-5]. In India, the fruits of the wild pomegranate have thicker rinds and extremely high acidity compared with cultivated types. They are also reported to have much smaller arils. In Central Asia, the primary difference noted is the higher acidity in wild material. The pomegranate's origin in proximity to the ancient cultures of the Mediterranean has provided a long, recorded history for pomegranate. Indeed, some have argued that the pomegranate is the "apple" of the biblical Garden of Eden, but this is disputed in a recent review. Pomegranate has been naturalized throughout the Mediterranean region. Edible pomegranates were cultivated in Persia (Iran) by 3000 BCE, and were also present in Jericho in modern-day Israel. By 2000 BCE, Phoenicians had established Mediterranean Sea colonies in North Africa, bringing pomegranates to modern-day Tunisia and Egypt. Around the same time, pomegranates become naturalized in western Turkey and Greece. The pomegranate continued to be dispersed around the globe, reaching China by 100 BCE. By 800 CE, the fruit was spread throughout the Roman Empire, including Spain. At the same time, it was known to be extensively cultivated in Central and southern India. By the early 1400s, the pomegranate had made its way to Indonesia. In the 1500s and 1600s, the Spanish introduced this species to Central America, Mexico, and South America. The first clear evidence that the pomegranate was in the area to become the United States was in the early 1700s, when they were grown in Spanish Florida and English Georgia. By 1770, the pomegranate made its way to the West Coast and was growing in the missions of California [6-10] (Figure 1).

Both the Arabic name for pomegranate (rumman) and the Hebrew name (rimmon) are reported to originate as "fruit of paradise," which provides abundant demonstration of its appreciation in these cultures. In startling contrast, it was considered by the Greeks to be the "fruit of the dead" and provided sustenance to the residents of Hades [11]. These two considerations may demonstrate the amazing breadth of the pomegranate's potential consumer base. The fruit's unique flavours, with sweetness often counterbalanced by acidity, makes pomegranate easy to appreciate by most who try it. In addition to their use as a fresh fruit or fruit juice, the juice of the pomegranate also contributes distinctive character to many Middle Eastern dishes, such as the Iranian fessenjan.

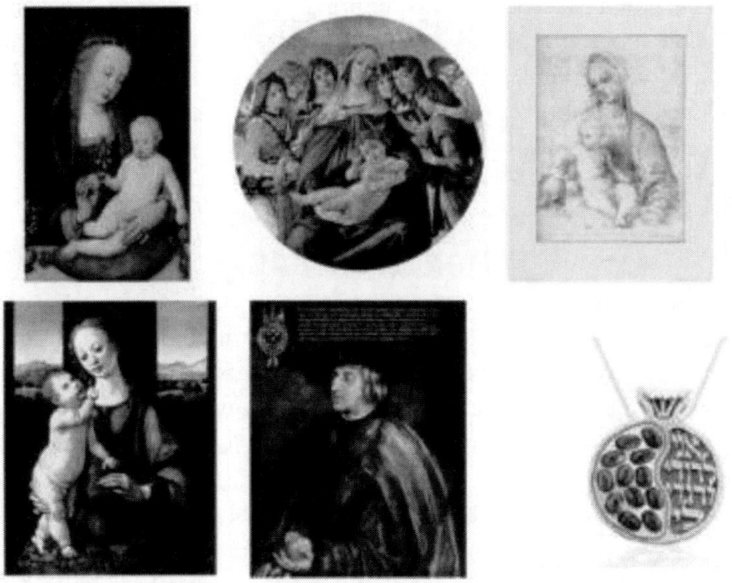

Figure 1. Works of art depicting pomegranate fruit, demonstrating the significance of this fruit in religion, culture, and society. First row, from left to right: "Maria, dem Kind einen Granatapfel reichend" by Hans Holbein the Elder, Boticelli's "Madonna of the Pomegranate" (1487), and Raphael's "Virgin and Child with Pomegranate". Second row, from left to right: Lorenzo Di Credi's "Madonna and Child with a Pomegranate (Dreyfus Madonna)", Albrecht Duerer's "Maximilian I of Habsburg", and a Jewish pendant.

As a practical contributor to the diet, these fruits were likely invaluable to early desert travellers as an easily carried, well protected form of water [11]. In Zoroastrianism, the pomegranate symbolizes both fecundity and immortality, and is an emblem of prosperity [12]. Pomegranate has long been associated with love and was one of the symbols of the love goddess Aphrodite. In the biblical Song of Songs, Sheba ecstatically replies to

Solomon's blandishments: "Let us get up early to the vineyards; let us see if the vine flourish, whether the tender grape appear, and the pomegranates bud forth: there will I give thee my love." Indeed Solomon describes Sheba as a garden whose "plants are an orchard of pomegranates" and says, "as a piece of a pomegranate are thy temples within thy locks." Sheba then says she wants Solomon to drink "the spiced wine of the juice of my pomegranate."

It is easy to imagine that the seediness of the pomegranate encouraged association with fertility. Perhaps this gave rise to the Greek myth in which Persephone must spend 6 months in the underworld after Hades forced her to eat six pomegranate seeds, but her return is celebrated with the coming of spring. A bit more mysterious is the rationale for Hebrew priests wearing vestments adorned with pomegranates (Exodus 28:31), or the 480 BCE attempt by King Xerxes to capture Greece with an army carrying spears adorned with pomegranates [12].

HORTICULTURE

The pomegranate plant inherently develops numerous trunks. In orchards, plants are normally trained to a single trunk, We acknowledge Matt Quist and Jason Haught, Paramount Farming Company; Zeev Wiesman, Institutes for Applied Research, Ben Gurion University of the Negev, Beer Sheva, Israel; Claudia Botti, Department of Agronomy, University of Santiago, Chile; and Londhe Santosh Dinkar and Dr. R.B. Sawant, College of Agriculture, Shivaji University, Kolhapur, India forming a large shrub or small tree, and reaching a height of 12 to 20 ft at maturity. Trees may be trained to multiple trunks in colder areas, to reduce risk of total tree loss. Very dwarf pomegranates (such as 'Nana') are known with small plant, flower, and fruit sizes, and are widely used as ornamentals. The pomegranate plant is more or less spiny and deciduous, with small, narrow, oblong leaves with short stems [13-14]. Plants aggressively sucker from the crown area and the roots. The pomegranate flowers are most commonly red to red–orange and are funnel shaped, although "double" and variegated flowers are found in some ornamental selections, which are not grown for fruit. Pomegranate can be self-pollinated or cross-pollinated by insects (Morton, 1987). Flowers are primarily borne sub terminally, primarily on short lateral branches older than 1 year (El- Kassas et al., 1998), although some cultivars flower on spurs. Flowers occur as single blossoms or in clusters of up to five. In the Central Valley of California, pomegranate blooms from early May to November, with most flowering from mid-May to early June. Pollination in California is primarily affected by insects or hummingbirds. Stigma receptivity lasts 2 to 3 d and declines quickly in unpollinated flowers [15-16].

Pomegranate flowers are heterostylous. Long-styled perfect flowers are larger, have larger ovaries, and set more fruit than short style types, which are either intermediate or functionally male only. The proportion of these two flower types varies among cultivars and year to year [17]. The pomegranate fruit is berrylike with a leathery rind (or husk) enclosing many seeds surrounded by the juicy arils, which comprise the edible portion of the fruit [18]. The aril juice sack is composed of many epidermal cells. According to cultivar, arils range from deep red to virtually colourless, whereas the enclosed seed varies in content of sclerenchyma tissue, which affects seed softness. The number of locules and arils (and enclosed seeds) varies, but may be as high as 1300 per fruit. The fruit has a prominent calyx, which is maintained to maturity and is a distinctive feature of the pomegranate fruit. The husk is comprised of two parts: the pericarp, which provides a cuticle layer and fibrous mat; and the mesocarp (known also as the albedo), which is the spongy tissue and inner fruit wall where the arils attach. Septal membranes are the papery tissue that further compartmentalizes groups of arils, but arils do not attach to this tissue (Matthew Quist, pers. comm.). There is interest in identifying or developing cultivars that have more locules to fill the fruit interior, fewer septal membranes for easier eating, and a thinner mesocarp [19].

Fruits ripen about 6 to 7 months after flowering [20] and are harvested when qualities are deemed most appropriate for expected market use. In Israel, they harvest 'Wonderful' when soluble solids reach 15% [21]. Minimum maturity for 'Wonderful' in California is based on titratable acidity less than 1.85% and colour darker than an established reference [21]. In a Spanish study, soluble solids of the cultivars examined did not vary greatly from mid-August through mid-November, and the principal acids were malic and citric [22].

Unlike most horticultural fruits, inherent seed dispersal is not achieved through consumption of all or most of the fruit and seeds with accompanying spread. Rather, the pomegranate fruit structure has apparently evolved to ensure splitting of the leathery husk, and exposure of the tempting arils and seeds [21] to the many happily cooperative birds and so forth serving as dispersal agents [23].

POMEGRANATE PRODUCTION

Current global production estimates for pomegranate are unavailable. However, it is widely grown in many countries where it is well adapted. In India more than 100,000 ha of pomegranate are produced. It is considered one of the most important fruits of the tropical and subtropical areas because of low maintenance cost, good yields, good keeping quality, and ability to thrive with limited moisture [24]. In Iran, 65,000 ha of pomegranate produce 600,000 tons of fruit annually, with about 30% of yield exported. Turkish production in 1997 was 56,000 tons/year. Spain, with 3000 ha, is the largest western European producer of pomegranates, and production has been increasing as a result of high market prices [25]. In the United States, there are 5600 ha of commercial pomegranate, mostly in the San Joaquin Valley. The 'Wonderful' cultivar dominates almost completely, but there is interest in earlier and later cultivars to extend the market season [26].

POMEGRANATE CULTIVARS

More than 500 cultivars of pomegranate have been named [27], but such ancient and widespread fruits often have considerable synonymy, in which the same basic genotype is known by different names in different regions. Synonymy is likely further encouraged by the fact that husk and aril colour can vary markedly when grown in different regions. A number of characteristics vary between pomegranate genotypes and are key to identification, consumer preference, preferred use, and potentially niche marketing. The most important traits are fruit size, husk colour (ranging from yellow to purple, with pink and red most common), aril colour (ranging from white to red), and hardness of the seed, maturity, juice content, acidity, sweetness, and astringency.

The 'Wonderful' cultivar was discovered in Florida and brought to California in 1896 [28]. This is the primary cultivar of commerce in the United States. It is also grown in Western Europe, Israel, and Chile [28]. 'Wonderful' is among the most deeply coloured of pomegranates in both husk and juice, with a rich flavour, good juice yield, and both sprightly acidity and slight thirst-quenching astringency similar to that of grapefruit juice and cranberries. Many pomegranate lovers consider it to be among the best-tasting cultivars. 'Wonderful' is nearly ideal for juicing, with excellent juice percentage as well as quality. It also has useful resistance to fruit cracking after rainfall on mature fruit. Other commercial U.S. cultivars include 'Granada' (a 'Wonderful' sport), 'Early Wonderful' (also a 'Wonderful' sport), and 'Early Foothill'. The cultivars 'Mollar de Elche' and 'Valenciana', in Spain, are among the most widely marketed pomegranate cultivars in Western Europe.

Table 1. Primary characteristics for pomegranate cultivars

Cultivar	Fruit size (g)	Traits	Origin
Agridulce de Ojós 4	524	Red arils with hard seeds, bitter/sweet, medium acid	Spain
Alandi (or Vadki)		Deep-pink arils and very hard seeds, sweet/sour	India
Asinar	505	Large fruit, red arils, sweet/sour, soft seeds	Turkey
Bedana		Medium-large, brownish white rind, pink–white arils, seeds soft, sweet	India
Borde de Albatera	370	Deep-red arils with hard seeds, bitter, high acid	Spain
Dholka		Large, yellow–red rind, white arils and hard seeds, sweet	India
Early Foothill		Deep-red arils, medium-hard seeds, sweet/sour	USA, 2–4 weeks earlier than 'Wonderful'
Early Wonderful		Deep-red arils, medium-hard seeds, sweet/sour	USA, 2 weeks earlier than 'Wonderful'
Eksilik		Sour (5% TA), red arils	Turkey
Emar		Dark-red skin, red arils, sweet with low TA	Turkey
Eversweet		Pink to red fruit with pink arils, soft, seeds, sweet even when immature	USA
Fellahyemez		Large pink arils, sweet with low TA, soft seeds	Turkey
Ganesh		Yellow–pink rind and pink–red arils, very soft seeds, sweet/sour	India
Golden Globe	"Very large"	Golden green fruit with pink blush, pink to red arils, soft, small seeds, sweet	USA
Granada		Deep-red arils, medium-hard seeds, sweet/sour	USA, redder, 1 month earlier sport of 'Wonderful'
Hicaznar		Dark-red skin, red arils, sweet/sour	Turkey
Kandhari (also called Arakta)		Large fruit, deep-red rind, with deep-pink to blood-red arils, hard seeds, sweet/sour	India
Katirbasi	517	Large fruit, large red arils, sweet/sour	Turkey
Mollar de Elche 15	272	Deep-red arils with soft seeds, sweet, low acid	Spain
Mollar de Orihuela	414	Red–pink arils with soft seeds, sweet, low acid	Spain
Piñón Tierno de Ojós 9	405	Red–pink arils with soft seeds, sweet, low acid	Spain
Valenciana		Small, early, but not top quality	Spain
Wonderful		Deep-red arils, medium-hard seeds (we would call medium-soft), sweet/sour	USA

The 'Valenciana' cultivar is harvested early (August),with very little sun damage and lower risk from pest attack or bad weather, but also has low yield, average to poor internal fruit quality, and small fruit size. The 'Mollar' cultivar is harvested much later (end of September until mid-November) and displays more sun and split damage, but has higher yield, excellent internal fruit quality, larger size, longer harvest period, and greater consumer acceptance [29].

Because of differences in quality and productivity observed in commercial plantings, Spanish researchers have selected distinct clones of their most important cultivars. Selections were made in 1986, in the provinces of Alicante and Murcia. Numbered clones were propagated and are undergoing replicated trials to identify the best materials [28].

The countries of pomegranate origin grow innumerable cultivars, with many regional favourites. Local pomegranate germplasm collections have been established in several Mediterranean countries, including Spain, Morocco, Tunisia, Greece, Turkey, and Egypt. India has three collections containing at least 30 accessions each. Azerbaijan, the Ukraine, Uzbekistan, and Tajikistan have collections of 200 to 300 accessions, and the collection of the Turkmenistan Experimental Station of Plant Genetic Resources is the largest in the world, containing more than 1000 accessions. The U.S. National Clonal Germplasm Repository, in Davis, CA, has almost 200 pomegranate accessions, including many obtained from the Turkmenistan collection. Included in this collection are several types with very soft seeds, a trait sometimes optimistically called "seedless." Interestingly, in a preliminary molecular marker study, genetic variability was found to be quite low among the diverse cultivars in the U.S. collection (M. Aradhya, pers. comm.). Little detailed information is available on pomegranates grown outside of Western Europe and the United States, although efforts have been made to assemble cultivar summary information for this paper (Table 1). Cultivars mentioned as important in the literature, but with no descriptions, include 'Ahmar', 'Aswad', and 'Halwa' from Iraq; 'Mangulati' from Saudi Arabia; and 'Red Loufani' and 'Ras el Baghl' from Israel and Palestine. Pomegranate cuttings root with great ease, facilitating spread of desirable clones. Efforts to graft pomegranate are reported not to be successful, but air-layering and root sucker transplantation can be used for vegetative propagation [30].

Pomegranate is especially well adapted to Mediterranean environments with cool winters and hot summers, but can be grown in the humid tropics or subtropics, and the plant will survive as far north as Washington, DC, but is injured by temperatures less than –11 °C [25]. Commercial production is concentrated in dry summer climates; a pomegranate is extremely drought tolerant once established, but crops much better with more generous moisture. Pomegranate thrives on a wide variety of soils and has a high resistance to salinity [26]. In all regions, newly planted trees require adequate moisture for establishment. For example, in California, plantings are established in late winter to spring when soil moisture is abundant from winter rain. Similarly plantings are made in India during the monsoon season (L.S. Dinkar, pers. comm.). Pomegranate cuttings root so easily that unrooted cuttings are sometimes placed directly into the orchard [15]. Plants are trained to one to five trunks and should receive light annual pruning to maintain the production of short spurs, which bear most fruit, and such pruning also reduces the potential for wind scarring on long whippy shoots.

Pomegranates will set a few fruit in the second or third year after propagation, but generally reach good commercial production at 5 to 6 years. When possible, providing adequate moisture is recommended throughout the growing season (with soil moistures similar to those used in citrus production), which contributes to growth, production, and a reduction in splitting [16]. It is especially important to avoid drought stress during initial fruit set. Pomegranate orchards benefit from 0.2 to 0.5 kg N/tree per year, applied once in fall or winter, or a split application in late winter and in spring.

High or late N application may compromise fruit maturity and colour. Zinc is the only other nutrient recommended for application to pomegranate in California. When Zn deficiency is evident, sprays should be applied to foliage in spring and early summer. Serious disease does not routinely affect pomegranate trees in California, but Alternaria heart rot, may sometimes affect fruit.

There are two widespread arthropod pests on commercial pomegranates in California: 1) the flat mite Brevipalpus lewisi and 2) the leafroller Platynola stultana. Both these pests cause rusting and checking on fruit. However, a number of species have caused localized damage in some years. In some other regions, Virachola species of moths are a severe threat and require multiple sprays each year [31]. This moth bores into the fruit, causing widespread fungal infections in the arils and bruising on the fruit surface. Premium prices for fresh fruit are obtained only for large blemish-free pomegranates. In India, developing fruit are sometimes protected from birds and other threats by bagging them on the tree [25]. Another practice in India is the "Mirg Bahar" practice of inducing drought stress from December through May so that the peak of production is in October and November [30]. Hand thinning is practiced in Israel to produce larger and more uniform fruit [31], and is also practiced in Spain. Storage life of the pomegranate is quite long and equals the apple, and the fruits ship very well, although bruising can be an issue. The pomegranate fruit is not climateric [32] Harvest and storage factors affecting postharvest quality of pomegranate have been summarized in a recent review [32].

MEDICINAL AND OTHER USES

According to Eber's papyrus (ca. 1550 BCE), the ancient Egyptians used tannin-rich pomegranate root extracts for the riddance of tapeworms [33]. Hippocrates (400 BCE) used pomegranate extractions for a wide variety of ailments, such as a plaster to reduce skin and eye inflammation, and as an aid to digestion [34]. No discussion of ancient medical applications of plants is complete without mention of Dioscorides (40–90 CE), who indicates: "All sorts of pomegranates are of a pleasant taste and good for ye stomach"and further suggests the juice for ulcers, and for ye paines of years, and for the griefs in ye nosthrills" [35]. Other traditional uses of pomegranate products have included treatments for contraception, snakebite, diabetes, and leprosy. Extracts of tannins (bark, leaves, and immature fruit) have been used to halt diarrhoea and haemorrhage, whereas dried; crushed flower buds are made into a tea as remedy for bronchitis. In Mexico, extracts of the flowers are used as a gargle to relieve mouth and throat inflammation [25]. Interestingly, many of these uses are at least somewhat supported by recent scientific studies [36]. However, it must be noted that there is no report of trials using pomegranate to treat snakebite. Presumably because of its association as the "fruit of love" rather than empirical observation, the pomegranate has been considered a love potion in some cultures. The prophet Mohammed advised, "Eat the pomegranate, for it purges the system of envy and hatred". Today, pomegranate juice has been shown to contain polyphenol antioxidants (primarily ellagic acid and punicalagin) that may lower risk of heart disease [37] and may slow cancer progress [38]. Largely because of the interest in health benefits of pomegranate, 40 journal publications were produced on this fruit in 2005 versus 30 totals from 1945 to 2000 [39].

There are a number of other useful applications for the product of the pomegranate tree. Pomegranate bark produces tannins that help create Moroccan leather. Extracts of the flowers and fruit husks have been used as dyes for textiles. Extracts of pomegranate rinds provided a major source of medieval ink in Europe [1-10], and specialty craft inks are still created from pomegranate. Clearly, the most widespread "non-food" use of pomegranate is for visual aesthetics. Several ornamental plant forms have been touched on already, and these are widespread in the nursery industry where pomegranate is adapted. The distinctive appearance and long life of the mature harvested pomegranate fruit results in their widespread use in table arrangements. In the United States, this is especially common during the Thanksgiving through Christmas season. The longstanding nature of this use is apparent from pomegranate's frequent inclusion in paintings and as graphic elements in architecture, for example. This visual aesthetic use is so widespread that most of the pomegranates purchased as fresh fruit in the United States are likely never actually consumed (California) [39-42].

FUTURE PROSPECTS AND CONCLUSION

Increased interest in phytonutrients appears likely to sustain and increase interest in pomegranate within the United States. 'Wonderful' juice is widely available in the refrigerated produce section of supermarkets and has displayed considerable sales growth. Numerous techniques are being explored to enhance postharvest life and quality of fresh pomegranate. Consumer reluctance to open and eat intact fruits, which some suggest is best "best performed naked, outdoors or in the bathtub" has encouraged development of methods to blow out arils and package these beautiful jewels as a minimally processed fresh product These will soon find their way to market and will likely be eaten as snacks and used as garnishes in salads and savoury dishes. The preference of some consumers for cultivars with less acid or softer seeds is also compelling consideration of more diverse cultivars, which should broaden consumer interest. When these "wonderful" properties are combined with a Food and Drug Administration label as a "love potion" and the prophet's prescription for curing "hatred and envy," it may be impossible to keep up with the demand for this amazing fruit.

REFERENCES

[1] Adams, F. 1849. *Genuine works of Hippocrates*. William Wood and Co., New York.

[2] Adams, L.S., N.P. Seeram, B.B. Aggarwal, Y. Takada, D. Sand, and D. Heber. 2006. Pomegranate juice, total pomegranate ellagitannins, and punicalagin suppress inflammatory cell signalling in colon cancer cells. *J. Agr. Food Chem.* 54:980–985.

[3] Amoros, A., P. Melgarejo, J.J. Martinez, F. Hernández, and M. Martinez. 2000. Characterization of the fruit of five pomegranate (Punica granatum L.) clones cultivated in homogeneous soils. *Options Méditerranéennes Ser. A* 42:129–135. Anarinco. 2006. Pomegranate history. 1 Sept. 2006. <www.anarainco.com/history.htm>.

[4] Artés, F. and F.A. Tomás-Barberán. 2000. Postharvest technological treatments of pomegranate and preparation of derived products. *Options Méditerranéennes Ser. A* 42:199–204.

[5] Aviram, M., M. Rosenblat, D. Gaitini, S. Nitecki, A. Hoffman, L. Dornfeld, N. Volkova, D. Presser, J. Attias, H. Liker, and T. Hayek. 2004. Pomegranate juice consumption for 3 years by patients with carotid artery stenosis reduces common carotid intima-media thickness, blood pressure and LDL oxidation. *Clin. Nutr.* 23:423–433.

[6] Bist, H.S., R. Srivastava, and G. Sharma. 1994. Variation in some promising selections of wild pomegranate (Punica granatum L.). *Hort. J.* 7:67–70.

[7] Blumenfeld, A., F. Shaya, and R. Hillel. 2000. Cultivation of pomegranate. *Options Méditerraneennes Ser. A* 42:143–147. California Rare Fruit Growers. 1997. Pomegranate. 1 Sept. 2006. <www.crfg.org /pubs/ff/pomegranate.html>.

[8] Carvalho, D.N. 1999. Forty centuries of ink. The World Wide School, Seattle, WA. 1 Sept. 2006. <www.worldwideschool.org/library/books/ tech/printing/FortyCenturiesofInk/chap7.html>.

[9] Costa, Y. and P. Melgarejo. 2000. A study of the production costs of two pomegranate varieties grown in poor quality soils. *Options Méditerranéennes Ser. A* 42:49–53.

[10] Dave Wilson Nursery. 2005. Pomegranate1 Sept. 2006. <www.davewilson.com/br40/br40_trees/ br40Pomegranate.html>.

[11] El-Kassas, S.E., A.M. El-Sese, A.M. El-Salhy, and A.A. Abadıá. 1998. Bearing habits in some pomegranate cultivars. *Assiut J. Agr. Sci.* 29:147–162.

[12] Gozlekci, S. and L. Kaynak. 2000. Investigations on pollen production and quality in some standard pomegranate (Punica granatum L.) cultivars. *Options Méditerranéennes Ser. A* 42:71–77.

[13] Graham, S.A., J. Hall, K. Sytsma, and S. Shi. 2005. Phylogenetic analysis of the Lythraceae based on four gene regions and morphology. *Int. J. Plant Sci.* 166:995–1017.

[14] Gulick, P. and D.H. Van Sloten. 1984. *Directory of germplasm collections. (6.1)- Tropical and subtropical fruits and nut trees.* IBPGR, Rome, Italy.

[15] Gunter, R.T. 1934. *The Greek herbal of Dioscorides*, p. 80–81, Oxford University Press, Oxford, UK.

[16] Guo, C.J., J.Y. Wei, J.J. Yang, Y.F. Li, J. Xu, and Y.G. Jiang. 2003. The antioxidant capacity of 66 vegetables and fruits: A comparative study. *Acta Nutrimenta Sinica* 25:203–207.

[17] Kader, A.A. 2006. Postharvest biology and technology of pomegranates, p. 211–220. In: Seeram N, Schulman R, Heber D, eds. *Pomegranates Ancient Roots to Modern Medicine.* Taylor and Francis, Boca Raton, FL.

[18] Kader, A.A., A. Chordas, and S.M. Elyatem. 1984. Responses of pomegranates to ethylene treatment and storage temperature. *California Agr.* 38:4–15.

[19] Karp, D. 2006. The pomegranate: For one and all. *Fruit Gardener* 38:8–12.

[20] Kerimov, A. 1934. Biochemical study of the subtropical fruit trees of *Azerbaijan. Bul. Appl. Bot.* 5:325–348.

[21] Kher, R. 1999. A note on the physico-chemical characters of the wild pomegranate (Punica protopunica L.). *Ann. Biol. Ludhiana* 15:231– 232.

[22] Kosenko, V.N. 1985. Palynomorphology of representatives of the family Punicaceae. Bot. Z. 70:39–41. (from abstract only). Kotkin, C. 2006. Pomegranates on parade. *Wine News.* 1 Sept. 2006. <www.thewine news.com/decjan0506/cuisine.asp>.

[23] Lansky, E., S. Shubert, and I. Neeman. 2000. Pharmacological and therapeutic properties of pomegranate. *Options Méditerranéennes Ser. A* 42:231–235.

[24] LaRue, J.H. 1980. Growing pomegranates in California. *DANR publication leaflet* 2459. 1 Sept. 2006. <http://fruitsandnuts.ucdavis.edu/ crops/ pomegranate_factsheet.shtml#b>.

[25] Legua, P., P. Melgarejo, M. Martinez, and F. Hernández. 2000. Evolution of sugars and organic acid content in three pomegranate cultivars (Punica granatum L.). *Options Méditerranéennes Ser. A* 42:99-104.

[26] Genofund of pomegranate in Turkmenistan. *Problems Desert Dev.* 3:84–89.

[27] Levin, G.M. 2006. *Pomegranate*. Texas A&M Press, College Station, TX.

[28] Mars, M. 2000. Pomegranate plant material: Genetic resources and breeding, a review. *Options Méditerranéennes Ser. A* 42:55–62.

[29] Martinez, J.J., P. Melgarejo, and F. Martinez. 2000. Study of the floral morphology of the pomegranate clones: PTO8, CRO1 and ME14. *Options Méditerranéennes Ser. A* 42:105– 113.

[30] McDonald, J.A. 2002. Botanical determination of the Middle Eastern tree of life. *Econ. Bot.* 56:113–129.

[31] Mehrnews. 2006. Iran, only producer of premium pomegranate. 1 Sept. 2006. <www.mehrnews. com/en/NewsDetail.aspx?NewsID=216517>.

[32] Melgarejo, P. 2003. *Tratado de fruticultura para zonas aridas y semoaridas. II. Algarrobo, granado y jinjolero*. Mundi-prensa, Madrid.

[33] Melgarejo, P., P. Legua, M. Martinez, and J.J. Martinez. 2000. Contribution to a better knowledge of the quality of pomegranate pollen (Punica granatum L.). *Options Méditerranéennes Ser. A* 42:115–121.

[34] Morton, J. 1987. *Fruits of warm climates*. Miami, FL.

[35] Panthaky, R.G.N. 2006. Significance of pomegranate tree in our religion. 1 Sept. 2006. <http:// tenets.zoroastrianism.com/pomen33. html>. POM Wonderful. 2006. 1 Sept. 2006. <www.pomwonderful. com>.

[36] Schulman, R.N. 2006. Summary, p. 223–226. In: N.P. Seeram, R.N. Schulman, and D. Heber (eds.). *Pomegranates: Ancient Roots to Modern Medicine*. CRC Press, Boca Raton, FL.

[37] Seelig, R.A. 1970. *Fruit & vegetable facts & pointers: Pomegranates*. United Fresh Fruit Association, Washington, DC.

[38] Seeram N.P., R.N. Schulman, and D. Heber (eds.). 2006. *Pomegranates: Ancient Roots to Modern Medicine*. CRC Press, Boca Raton, FL.

[39] Sepulveda, E., L. Galleti, C. Saenz, and M. Tapia. 2000. Minimal processing of pomegranate var. Wonderful. *Options Méditerranéennes Ser. A* 42:237–242.

[40] Shilikina, I.A. 1973. On the xylem anatomy of the genus Punica L. *Bot. Z.* 58:1628–1630. (access to abstract only).

[41] Still, D.W. 2006. Pomegranates: A botanical perspective, p. 199–209 In: Seeram N, Schulman R, Heber D, eds. *Pomegranates Ancient Roots to Modern Medicine*. Taylor and Francis, Boca Raton, FL.

[42] Schulman, and D. Heber (eds.). *Pomegranates: Ancient Roots to Modern Medicine*. CRC Press, Boca Raton, FL.

[43] Watson, L. and M.J. Dallwitz. 1992. *The families of flowering plants: Descriptions, illustrations, identification, and information retrieval.* 1 Sept. 2006. <http://delta-intkey.com>.

[44] Wren, R.C. 1988. *Potter's new cyclopedia of botanical drugs and preparations*. C.W. Daniel, Essex, UK.1092.

Chapter 2

CULTIVATION AND PRODUCTION OF POMEGRANATES

ABSTRACT

Various aspects of pomegranate cultivation will be discussed in this chapter. Tradition, consumption and production target, recommended soil, fertilisation and fertirrigation, most common diseases and treatments, weed control, tree shape and orchard design, pruning, preharvest treatment of fruits, harvesting, packing, storage and needs for the future will also be mentioned.

INTRODUCTION

Pomegranate has been mentioned in the Bible and has been included in which Israel's practices and traditions for centuries. It grew in the Holy land for thousands of years and is very much adapted to it: it sheds its leaves in the cold of our winters, while it sprouts in early spring when temperatures rise. It ripens at the end of the summer, very close to the beginning of the Jewish New Year. It was and is used for decoration and blessings in ceremonies of the New Year celebrations and the later holidays. It decorated temples in the past and appeared on ancient coins [1-4].

Owing to its decorative nature in Israel, its selection was done mainly for external appearance, rather than for eating quality. Its luscious colour and crown are very important characteristics of the fruit (Figure 1). Pomegranates are not distinguished by their names in Israel and price is based largely on appearance [4]. Some pomegranates have a hard rind with a bitter yellow diaphragm. These juices typically stain hands and clothes. Therefore "tools" are required to prepare the fruit for eating. Other pomegranate varieties can be eaten directly [4-6].

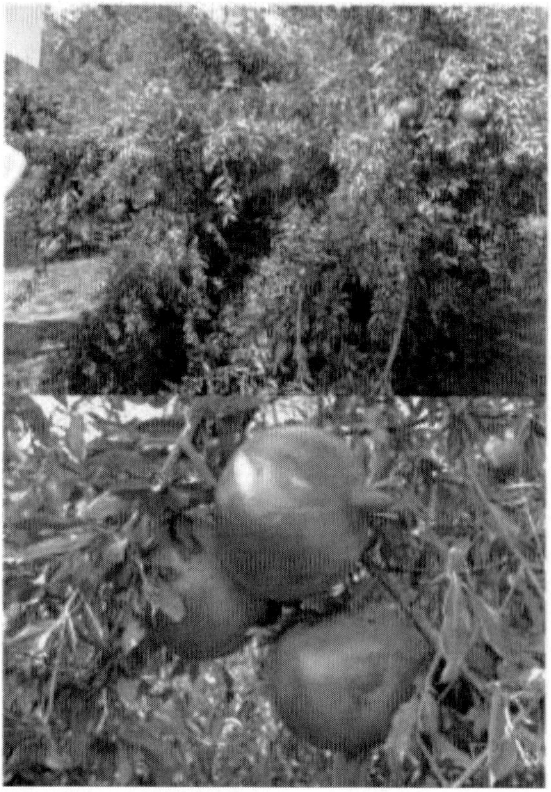

Figure 1. Pomegranate fruit and orchard.

Historically, pomegranates were cultivated in Israel in mixed orchards like many other trees. Nowadays, they still grow this way but are also available in home gardens worldwide. Pomegranates can be cultivated in uniform blocks of 1-5 hectares size, using modern technology. The aim of the growers is to produce more than 30 tons per hectare of high quality fruits. Larger fruits obtain higher prices than small ones. Fruit weight should exceed 400 grams. Best fruits should have nice colour, preferably red with a nice crown. Grains should be pink-red, large, and sweet with pleasant aroma [6-13]. The seeds should be soft.

SOILS

Pomegranate can be successfully grown in all soils except those that are calcareous or saline [13-17]. Orchards in Israel have medium or heavy soils with optimal drainage. In heavy soils ridges are sometimes prepared to have a better aeration of the root system in order to obtain higher production. Light-sandy soils are satisfactory if they are regularly irrigated.

The shape and size of the mature trees affects the orchard design. Generally in Israel the trees are standing alone, producing all around the tree [14-15]. No hedges are created. As the planting material of pomegranate is very cheap, there is a tendency to overcrowd the orchard. In a crowded orchard, production is lowered, fruits are set only at the top of the trees, colouring is bad and distribution of spraying materials is very bad [16].

TREE SHAPE

New branches are left one per trunk in order to renew old trunks. The light penetration from between the rows depends on the distance between the rows and on the height of the trees [17]. Taller trees will be more expensive to harvest as fruits will be mostly at the top of the trees.

Table 1. Effect of irrigation treatments on total soluble solids (TSS), titratable acidity (TA), maturity index (MI), and CIE L*, a* and b* colour coordinates at the eight picking times. Means within a column for each harvest that do not have a common letter are significantly different by LSD0.05 test. C*, chroma; H◦, hue angle

		Day of the year (DOY)							
Parameter	Treatment	236	252	264	287, harvest I	295, harvest II	301	307, harvest III	315
TSS (°Brix)	T0	12.3^{a}	14.1^{b}	14.8^{b}	16.4^{a}	16.2^{b}	16.1^{b}	16.2^{a}	16.4^{b}
	T1	13.6^{a}	15.7^{a}	16.3^{a}	17.2^{a}	17.6^{a}	17.6^{a}	17.9^{a}	18.3^{a}
TA (g citric acid 100 g^{-1})	T0	0.23^{a}	0.19^{b}	0.20^{a}	0.26^{a}	0.20^{a}	0.23^{a}	0.25^{a}	0.26^{a}
	T1	0.20^{b}	0.20^{a}	0.20^{a}	0.21^{a}	0.23^{a}	0.23^{a}	0.25^{a}	0.26^{a}
MI (TSS/TA)	T0	47.8^{a}	75.9^{a}	74.8^{b}	62.9^{b}	80.9^{a}	70.1^{a}	65.1^{b}	64.2^{b}
	T1	68.6^{a}	77.0^{a}	82.4^{a}	81.3^{a}	76.7^{a}	71.3^{a}	72.0^{a}	69.9^{a}
L^*	T0	67.2^{a}	72.1^{a}	73.9^{a}	70.5^{a}	72.3^{a}	68.8^{a}	63.8^{a}	65.3^{a}
	T1	67.7^{a}	70.3^{b}	74.2^{a}	60.8^{b}	59.9^{b}	54.3^{b}	52.7^{b}	48.0^{b}
a^*	T0	-6.2^{a}	-2.9^{b}	8.1^{b}	29.8^{b}	26.9^{b}	27.8^{b}	35.1^{b}	28.0^{b}
	T1	-9.8^{a}	2.1^{a}	12.4^{a}	40.4^{a}	43.8^{a}	45.2^{a}	44.6^{a}	42.0^{a}
b^*	T0	43.3^{a}	45.8^{a}	44.0^{a}	35.7^{a}	35.7^{a}	34.0^{a}	27.5^{a}	26.7^{a}
	T1	44.3^{a}	42.6^{b}	42.9^{a}	30.5^{b}	29.0^{b}	23.3^{b}	21.3^{b}	18.7^{b}
C^*	T0	43.9^{a}	46.0^{a}	44.7^{a}	47.5^{a}	44.8^{b}	43.9^{a}	44.7^{a}	38.8^{b}
	T1	45.5^{a}	42.8^{b}	44.9^{a}	51.1^{a}	52.0^{a}	50.9^{a}	49.3^{a}	45.9^{a}
$H°$	T0	98.1^{a}	93.6^{a}	82.1^{a}	50.9^{a}	53.0^{a}	50.7^{a}	38.0^{a}	43.9^{a}
	T1	102^{b}	87.1^{a}	73.9^{b}	37.6^{b}	32.7^{b}	27.2^{b}	25.8^{b}	24.0^{b}

Pruning orchards in winter helps to achieve the desired shape of trees [18]. This allows the height of the tree to be maintained at the desired height, whilst broken, bent, and interfering branches are removed. Summer pruning is necessary to keep the interior of the tree open during growing season [19-20].

Irrigation is necessary to maintain growth and wash away the pesticides (Table 1). Orchards should be irrigated twice a week and this allows the roots which are closer to the surface to grow and enhance fruit production. The amount of irrigation per day is dependent on the climate [19-20].

FERTIRRIGATION

Fertilisers are supplied to the orchard via the irrigation system. A typical orchard requires up to 200-300 kg/hectare nitrogen and potassium (K_2O) annually. Phosphoric acid is sued to clean the drip irrigation [21].

Unlike most other fruit trees pomegranate orchards are seldom manured. Rotten organic manure is sometimes added below the dripper lines by a few cultivators; however, it is thought that this practice slows down root growth. Commercial cultivation of pomegranate is required to help protect plants against a variety of fruit insects (Table 2). Fruits are susceptible to infection if they are not treated well. Therefore, pomegranate orchards are generally sprayed every 10-14 days with organic phosphor compounds which are gradually replaced by consecutive sprays [22-25].

Table 2. Insects that induce potential damage to pomegranate plants

Scientific name	Damage	Treatment
Virachola livia	Fruit. Grains rotting	Organic phosphates
Criptoblabos gnidiella	Fruit crown rotting in storage	Insecticide spray every 10-14 days Diazinon B.T.
Planococcus citri	Fruit crown, appearance	
Aphis punica	Growth inhibition of young trees	Dimecron
Tenupalpus granati	Leaves drop	Miticides
Enzophera sp.	Girdling root crown. Severe decline of trees	

Young plants are generally infected by aphids. While in mature orchards fruit sprays kill the aphids, a considerable addition of growth was obtained in young orchards by treating with "Confidur" (Imidacloprid). The spread of weed is regulated only by mowing, while nets are placed over the orchards. However, shading by the nets may reduce flower differentiation and fruit yields [26].

Preharvest Treatments of Fruit

In order to obtain fruits without damage to the rind and with good colour, some farmers clean the small branches around the fruits which might scratch the fruit. By doing this they also expose the fruit to sunlight. There is an idea to use reflective plastic sheets underneath the foliage to improve colour.

Physiological Disorders

The main disorder which causes a severe economic impact is splitting of ripe fruit [27-30]. The damage can be even of half of the yield. Some growers claim that if they leave more fruits on a tree the phenomena are larger, and that thinning helps to reduce it. Another explanation is that when they leave more fruits per tree and wait for it to attain regular size, the grains swell and crack the rind. Another form of damage is sunburn on fruit rind which reduces its value. The damage happens only at a certain physiological stage of fruit development.

Harvesting

As mentioned before, more than in other fruits, pomegranates are used for decorative purposes [30-34]. Therefore the most important criteria for beginning of harvesting are the external appearance, mainly the colour but also the "fullness" of the fruit. After careful observation of external appearance fruits are packed according to size in 2½ kg card boxes for export and around 8 kg for the local market. When supply is bigger than the demand, and for prolonging the season, fruits can be stored in cold storage. Fruits are kept at 7°C and 90% R.h. Only clean fruits with no insect damage, especially clear of criptoblabos gnidiella damages, are stored. Fruits damaged by the insect may rot in storage. Fruits can be easily stored for a period of 3 months. If the stored fruit is not mature, external browning of the rind occur [30-34]. Pomegranates can be stored in the ambient conditions for quite a long time. The rind dries and turns brown but the inside grains are kept well.

FUTURE PROSPECT AND CONCLUSION

In many countries, the pomegranate which is a traditional crop, or a new crop, needs more Investment in research and development. In order to base the knowledge on sound ground, such are the needs for fertilising, for irrigation and for other horticultural practices (Figure 2).

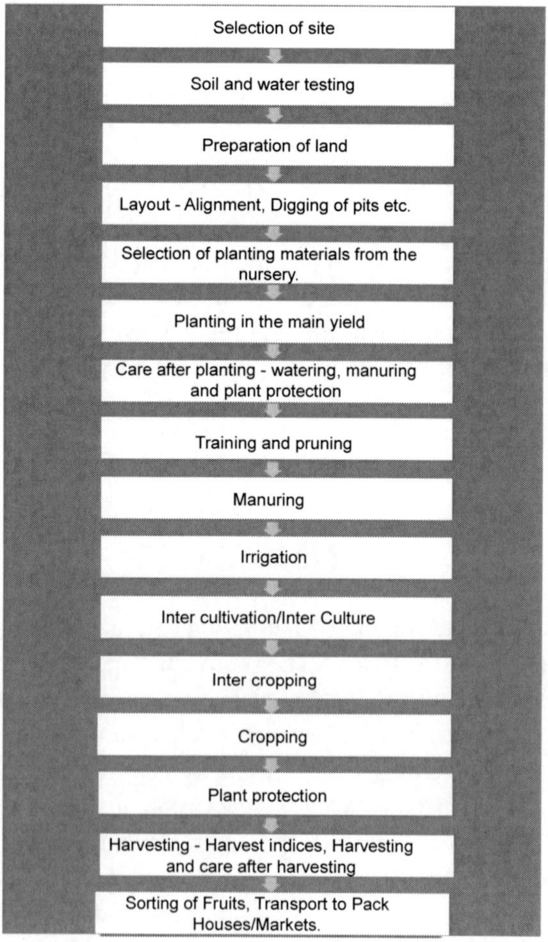

Figure 2. Flowchart for Pomegranate cultivation.

More environmentally-friendly plant protection practices have to be developed, as the markets demand cleaner (from pesticides) fruits, than it obtains today. Better cultivars, of higher internal quality of fruits, have to be cultivated. Standards of quality are needed in the markets. Cooperation in research, development and exchange of the existing knowledge are some of the first steps towards better production and products.

REFERENCES

[1] Melgarejo P, Salazar DM and Artés F, Organic acids and sugars composition of harvested pomegranate fruits. *Eur Food Res Technol* 211:185–190 (2000).

[2] Basu A and Penugonda K, Pomegranate juice: A heart-healthy fruit juice. *Nutr Rev* 67:49–56 (2009).

[3] Malik A, Afaq F, Sarfaraz S, Adhami V, Syed D and Mukhtar H, Pomegranate fruit juice for chemoprevention and chemotherapy of prostate cancer. *Proc Natl Acad Sci USA* 102:14813–14818 (2005).

[4] Aviram M and Dornfeld L, Pomegranate juice consumption inhibits serum angiotensin converting enzyme activity and reduces systolic blood pressure. *Atherosclerosis* 158:195–198 (2001).

[5] Sumner MD, Elliott-Eller M, Weidner G, Daubenmier JJ, Chew MH and Marlin R, Effects of pomegranate juice consumption on myocardial perfusion in patients with coronary heart disease. *Am J Cardiol* 96:810–814 (2005).

[6] Stover E and Mercure EW, The pomegranate: A new look at the fruit of paradise. *HortScience* 42:1088–1092 (2007).

[7] Holland D, Hatib K and Bar-Yàakov I, Pomegranate: botany, horticulture, breeding. *Hort Rev* 35:127–191 (2009).

[8] MAGRAMA, Ministerio de Agricultura, Alimentacin y Medio Ambiente. Anuario de Estadística Agraria 2012 Available: http://www.magrama.gob.es/estadistica/pags/anuario/2012/AE_2012_Completo. pdf [30 September 2013]

[9] Rodríguez P, Mellisho CD, Conejero W, Ortuño MF, Cruz ZN, Galindo A, et al., Plant water relations of leaves of pomegranate trees under different irrigation conditions. *Environ Exp Bot* 77:19–24 (2012).

[10] Aseri GK, Jain N, Panwar J, Rao AV and Meghwal PR, Biofertilizers improve plant growth, fruit yield, nutrition, metabolism and rhizosphere

enzyme activities of pomegranate (*Punica granatum* L.) in Indian Thar Desert. *Sci Hort* 117:130–135 (2008).
[11] Sarkhosh A, Zamani Z, Fatahi R and Ebadi A, RAPD markers reveal polymorphism among some Iranian pomegranate (*Punicagranatum* L.) genotypes. *Sci Hort* 111:24–29 (2006).
[12] Mellisho CD, Egea I, Galindo A, Conejero W, Rodríguez P, Rodríguez J, et al., Pomegranate (*Punica granatum* L.) fruit response to different deficit irrigation conditions. *Agric Water Manage* 114:30–36 (2012).
[13] Mena P, Galindo A, Collado-González J, Ondoño S, García-Viguera C, Ferreres F, et al., Sustained deficit irrigation affects the colour and phytochemical characteristics of pomegranate juice. *J Sci Food Agric* 93:1922–1927 (2013).
[14] Koppel K, Chambers IV E, Vázquez-Araújo L, Timberg L, Carbonell-Barrachina AA and Suwonsichon S, Cross-country comparison of pomegranate juice acceptance in Estonia, Spain, Thailand, and United States. *Food Qual Prefer* 31:116–123 (2014).
[15] Calín-Sánchez A, Martínez JJ, Vázquez-Araújo L, Burló F, Melgarejo P and Carbonell-Barrachina AA, Volatile composition and sensory quality of Spanish pomegranates (*Punica granatum* L.). *J Sci Food Agric* 91:586–592 (2011).
[16] Allen RG, Pereira RS, Raes D and Smith M, *Crop Evapotranspiration – Guidelines for Computing Crop Water Requirements*, v. 56, FAO Irrigation and Drainage 56. Food and Agriculture Organization, Rome (1998).
[17] Singleton VL, Orthofer R and Lamuela-Raventos RM, Analysis of total phenols and other oxidation substrates and antioxidants by means of Folin–Ciocalteu reagent. *Methods Enzymol* 299:152–178 (1999).
[18] Giusti MM, Rodriguez-Saona LE and Wrolstad RE, Molar absorptivity and color characterisque of acylated and non-acylated pelargodine based anthocyanins. *J Agric Food Chem* 47:4631–4637 (1999).
[19] Egea MI, Sánchez-Bel P, Marínez-MadridMC, Flores FB and Romojaro F, The effect of beta ionization on the antioxidant potential of 'Búlida' apricot and its relationship with quality. *Post Biol Technol* 46:63–70 (2007).
[20] Hale MG and Orcutt DM, *The Physiology of Plants Under Stress*. Wiley, New York (1987).
[21] Tehranifara A, Zareia M, Nematia Z, Esfandiyaria B and Vazifeshenas MR, Investigation of physico-chemical properties and antioxidant

activity of twenty Iranian pomegranate (*Punica granatum* L.) cultivars. *Sci Hort* 126:180–185 (2010).

[22] Shwartz E, Glazer I, Bar-Ya'akov I, Matityahu I, Bar-Ilan I, Holland D, et al., Changes in chemical constituents during the maturation and ripening of two commercially important pomegranate accessions. *Food Chem* 115:965–973 (2009).

[23] Kulkarni AP and Aradhya SM, Chemical changes and antioxidant activity in pomegranate arils during fruit development. *Food Chem* 93:319–324 (2005).

[24] Al-Maiman SA and Ahmad D, Changes in physical and chemical properties during pomegranate (*Punica granatum* L.) fruit maturation. *Food Chem* 76:437–441 (2002).

[25] Fawole OA and Opara UL, Changes in physical properties, chemical and elemental composition and antioxidant capacity of pomegranate (cv. Ruby) fruit at five maturity stages. *Sci Hort* 150:37–46 (2013).

[26] Laribi AI, Palou L, Intrigliolo DS, Nortes PA, Rojas-Argudo C, Taberner V, et al., Effect of sustained and regulated deficit irrigation on fruit quality of pomegranate cv. 'Mollar de Elche' at harvest and during cold storage. *Agric Water Manage* 125:61–70 (2013).

[27] Dixon J, Temperature and atmosphere composition influence on colour change of apples. MS thesis, Massey University, Palmerston North, New Zealand (1993).

[28] Hernández F, Melgarejo P, Tomás-Barberán FA and Artés F, Evolution of juice anthocyanins during ripening of newselectedpomegranate (*Punica granatum*) clones. *Eur Food Res Technol* 210:39–42 (1999).

[29] Zarei M, Azizi M and Bashir-Sadr Z, Evaluation of physicochemical characteristics of pomegranate (*Punica granatum* L.) fruit during ripening. *Fruits* 66:121–129 (2011).

[30] Shulman Y, Fainberstein L and Lavee S, Pomegranate fruit development and maturation. *J Hort Sci Biotechnol* 59:265–274 (1984).

[31] Mena P, Garcia-Viguera C, Navarro-Rico J, Moreno DA, Bartual J, Saura D, et al., Phytochemical characterization for industrial use of pomegranate (*Punica granatum* L.) cultivars grown in Spain. *J Sci Food Agric* 91:1893–1906.

[32] Fischer UA, Carle R and Kammerer DR, Identification and quantification of phenolic compounds from pomegranate (*Punica granatum* L.) peel, mesocarp, aril and differently produced juices by HPLCDAD– ESI/MSn. *Food Chem* 127:807–821 (2011).

[33] Borochov-Neori H, Judeinstein S, Tripler E, Harari M, Greenberg A, Shomer I, et al., Seasonal and cultivar variations in antioxidant and sensory quality of pomegranate (*Punica granatum* L.) fruit. *J Food Comp Anal* 22:189–195 (2009).

[34] Collado-González J, Cruz ZN, Rodríguez P, Galindo A, Díaz-Baños FG, García de la Torre J, et al., Effect of water deficit and domestic storage on the procyanidin profile, size, and aggregation process in pear-jujube (*Z. jujube*) fruits. *J Agric Food Chem* 61:6187–6197 (2013).

Chapter 3

FLAVOUR OF POMEGRANATES

ABSTRACT

Despite the recently discovered health-promoting benefits of pomegranates, relatively little is known regarding its sensory quality and flavor preferences, or about the biochemical constituents that determine its sensory characteristics. The present chapter we will discuss the sensory quality and flavor preferences of pomegranate fruit, including the genetic diversity in flavor characteristics among distinct varieties. Additionally, the dynamic changes that occur in fruit flavor during fruit ripening and postharvest storage will also be described briefly.

INTRODUCTION

The flavor of pomegranate fruit is perceived as a combination of basic taste, aroma and mouth feel sensations, by the brain during consumption of the food [1]. Taste, which comprises sweet, sour, bitter, salty and umami attributes, is detected by receptors located on the tongue and in the mouth that bind soluble components of the food matrix. In contrast, the sense of aroma is perceived via receptors present in the olfactory bulb in the nose cavity. These unique receptors specifically bind thousands of different volatiles. The sensory quality and biochemical constituents involved in creating the unique flavor of pomegranate fruit and juice, with special emphasis on flavor attributes of pomegranate arils will be discussed herein [1-10].

Sensory Attributes

Pomegranate juice is generally described as providing sweet and sour taste, musty/earthy and fruity odors, and an astringent mouth feel. Additional defined flavors were brown spice, fermented, molasses, vinegar, wine-like, woody, apple, berry, cranberry, cherry, grape, beet and carrot [11]. One study evaluated consumer satisfaction with various nutraceutically rich juices. The outcome of this study showed that the sensory attributes associated with pure pomegranate juice were beet, carrot, musty/earthy, fermented, sour cherry, other berries, bitter, throat burn, cranberry, prickle bite, tooth-etch, sour, astringency, skin/seeds and metallic flavors. Furthermore, it was indicated that astringency and bitterness attributes were classed as negative drivers of overall consumer liking of pomegranate juice [12-13].

In another recent study that specifically evaluated the flavor attributes of fresh pomegranate arils, with the aid of a trained descriptive sensory panel, it was reported that the overall flavor of pomegranate arils was a consequence of a combination of various taste (sweet, sour, bitter), aroma (red wine and pomegranate fruity notes) and mouth feel (astringency, juiciness and seed hardness) sensations. Furthermore, it was found that highly preferred pomegranate varieties were characterized by having high sweetness, moderate to low acidity levels, rich red wine and pomegranate fruity odors, low bitterness and astringency, and, preferably, soft seeds. In contrast, varieties with low flavor preference scores were found to be too sour or bitter, to have low red wine and pomegranate fruity odors, or to have very hard seeds [13].

Taste Components

The taste of pomegranate fruit mainly results from sensations of 'sweetness' and 'sourness' attributes. The sensation of 'sweetness' is governed by the presence of sugars, of which the most abundant molecules present in pomegranate juice are glucose and fructose; there are also minor amounts of other sugars such as sucrose, maltose and arabinose [14-16]. The sensation of 'sourness' in pomegranates is dependent on the presence of acids. Citric and malic acids are the two main acidic constituents. Other acids found in pomegranates include succinic, oxalic, tartaric and ascorbic acids. In addition to sweetness and sourness, pomegranates also exhibit a 'bitter' taste that results from the presence of high polyphenol contents. The bitter attribute is not very dominant in separated arils, but rather it could present a more serious problem in mechanically pressed pomegranate juice, because during the juice-manufacturing process polyphenol substances, which are present at high levels in the peel and capillary membranes, would be introduced into the squeezed, processed juice and enhance its bitterness. During the ripening process, pomegranate fruits undergo various biochemical changes leading to decreases in acid contents. These ripening-associated changes affect flavor perception, as early-season fruits are sourer than late-season ones [17-19].

The perceived taste of pomegranate fruit is also influenced by environmental and climatic conditions. Overall, it was demonstrated that in hot, dry desert climates pomegranate fruits accumulate lower acidity levels than those grown in a cooler Mediterranean climate. Indeed, most local pomegranate varieties grown in hot climates, such as those of India, Tunisia and Morocco, are considered 'sweet' and have very low acidity levels of between 1 and 4 g kg^{-1}. In contrast, pomegranate varieties native to colder regions, such as Turkey, Croatia and Georgia, are sourer and contain higher acidity levels of 9–43 g kg^{-1} [20-24].

AROMA

The aroma of pomegranate fruits is due to mixtures of dozens of volatiles belonging to diver's chemical classes. These volatiles present in pomegranates comprise three alcohols, six aldehydes, one ketone and 11 terpenes (six monoterpenes, two oxygenated terpenes and three sesquiterpenes) (Table 1) [25-38].

There is not just a single key character-impact compound accounting for the typical pomegranate odor; rather, the aroma of pomegranate fruits derives from a mixture of various volatiles that contribute 'green', 'woody', 'earthy', 'fruity', 'floral', 'sweet' and 'musty' notes. These aroma-active pomegranate volatiles include one ester, three aldehydes, five terpenes, two alcohols and one furan.

Table 1. Consensus aroma volatiles identified in fresh pomegranate juice

Compound	RI	Odour description	References
Alcohols (3)			
Hexanol	851	Resin, flower, green	24, 33–35, 37–38
(*Z*)-3-Hexenol	1039	Moss, fresh	24, 33–38
2-Ethylhexanol	1510	Floral	24, 35, 37
Aldehydes (6)			
Hexanal	801	Grass, tallow, fat	24, 33–38
(*E*)-2-Hexenal	844	Green, leaf	33–34, 38
Heptanal	903	Fat, citrus, rancid	24, 35–36
Octanal	999	Rancid, soapy	24, 35–38
Nonanal	1104	Fat, citrus, green	24, 33–34, 36–38
(*Z*)-3-Hexenal	1154	Green	33–34, 37
Ketones (1)			
6-Methyl-5-heptene-2-one	985	Oil, herbaceous, green	24, 34, 36–38
Monoterpenes (6)			
α-Pinene	939	Pine, turpentine	24, 33–34, 36
β-Pinene	981	Pine, resin, turpentine	24, 33–37
a-Terpinene	1012	Lemon	33–35
p-Cymene	1027	Solvent, citrus	34, 37–38
Limonene	1033	Lemon, orange	24, 33–34, 36–38
γ-Terpinene	1074	Gasoline, turpentine	24, 34, 38
Oxygenated monoterpenes (2)			
4-Terpineol	1179	Turpentine, must	24, 33, 36–38
α-Terpineol	1195	Oil, anise, mint	24, 33–34, 36–38
Sesquiterpenes (3)			
α-Bergamotene	1431	Wood, warm, tea	24, 36–37
β-Caryophyllene	1467	Wood, spice	24, 34–38

ASTRINGENCY

Astringency is a dry, puckering mouth feel sensation that can be elicited by eating unripe fruits that contain hydrolysable tannins, which bind to the salivary proteins, causing them to precipitate or aggregate and leading to a rough 'sandpapery' or dry sensation in the mouth. The major hydrolysable tannin present in pomegranate fruits, and responsible for the sensation of astringent mouth feel, is punicaligin, which is followed by smaller amounts of other hydrolysable tannins, such as gallic acid, ellagic acid and punicalin. In addition, phenolic compounds are also present in the seeds, from which they may be introduced into the juice. Thus high levels of hydrolysable tannins may impair overall consumer sensory satisfaction with the product [39-42].

Seed Hardness

Seed hardness is an important sensory attribute of pomegranate fruits grown for fresh consumption: the seeds can be difficult to chew and therefore impair consumer satisfaction. The seed hardness trait is usually measured according to the woody portion index (WPI), which represents the ratio of the woody portion of the seed to the entire aril [43-45].

Off Flavours

Fresh pomegranate fruits are stored in cold temperatures for at least a few weeks during the postharvest export and transportation processes. Some pomegranate varieties are often stored under controlled atmosphere or modified atmosphere conditions for up to 5 months after harvest. Long storage periods can lead to the development of off-flavors and impair sensory quality. The off-flavor is attributed to the accumulation of the ethanol fermentation products ethanol and ethyl acetate and of various sesquiterpene volatiles on the one hand, and the decrease in fruit flavor preference on the other. According to these evaluations, it seems that, in order to maintain flavor quality and reduce accumulation of off-flavors as far as possible, it is still necessary to optimize the postharvest storage protocols used for prolonged storage of pomegranate fruits [46].

Future Prospect and Conclusion

Along with the recent increase in global trading and demand for pomegranate as an important nutraceutical-rich fruit, for both fresh consumption and juice manufacturing, it became essential to fundamentally investigate pomegranate flavor quality, and to learn how various pre- and postharvest factors may influence the fruit's sensory quality and consumer acceptability. There is great importance to the genetic background of each pomegranate variety; in general, pomegranate fruit can be categorized according to total acidity levels into three major classes: 'sweet', 'sweet-sour' and 'sour' varieties. Accordingly, it is still necessary to optimize postharvest storage and transport conditions in order to maintain sensory quality and to reduce accumulation of off-flavor volatiles during storage and marketing.

REFERENCES

[1] Holland D, Hatib K and Bar-Ya'akov I, Pomegranate: botany, horticulture, breeding. *Hortic Rev* 35:127–191 (2009).

[2] Ozguven AL, Yilmaz C and Keles D, Pomegranate biodiversity and horticultural management. *Acta Hortic* 940:21–27 (2012).

[3] Stover E and Mercure EW, The pomegranate: a new look at the fruit of paradise. *Hort Science* 42:1088–1092 (2007).

[4] Still DW, Pomegranates: a botanical perspective, in *Pomegranates: Ancient Roots to Modern Medicine*, ed. by Seeram NP, Schulman RN and Heber D. CRC Press, Boca Raton, FL, pp. 211–222 (2006).

[5] Viuda-Martos M, Fernández-López J and Pérez-Álvarez JA, Pomegranate and its many functional components as related to human health: a review. *Comp Rev Food Sci Food Safety*

[6] Johanningsmeier SD and Harris GK, Pomegranate as a functional food and nutraceutical source. *Annu Rev Food Sci Technol* 2:181–201 (2011).

[7] Facial A and Ocalhau CA, The bioactivity of pomegranate: impact on health and disease. *Crit Rev Food Sci Nutr* 51:626–634 (2011).

[8] Rymon D, Mapping features of the global pomegranate market. *Acta Hortic* 890:599–602 (2011).

[9] Goff SA and Klee HJ, Plant volatile compounds: sensory cues for health and nutritional value? *Science* 311:815–819 (2006).

[10] Schwab W, Davidovich-Rikanati R and Lewinsohn E, Biosynthesis of plant-derived flavor compounds. *Plant J* 54:712–732 (2008).

[11] Koppel K and Chambers E, Development and application of a lexicon to describe the flavor of P omegranate Juice. *Journal of Sensory Studies* 25: 819-837.

[12] Lawless LJR, Threlfall RT, Meullenet JF and Howard LR, Applying a mixture design for consumer optimization of black cherry, concord grape and pomegranate juice blends. *J Sensory Stud* 28:102–112 (2013).

[13] Mayuoni-Kirshinbaum L, Bar-Ya'akov I, Hatib K, Holland D and Porat R, Genetic diversity and sensory preference in pomegranate fruits. *Fruits* (in press).

[14] Melgarejo P, Domingo MS and Artes F, Organic acids and sugar composition of harvested pomegranate fruits. *Eur Food Res Technol* (2000) 211:185-190.

[15] Dafny-Yalin M, Glazer I, Bar-Ilan I, Kerem Z, Holland D and Amir R, Color, sugars and organic acids composition in aril juices and peel homogenates prepared from different pomegranate accessions. *J Agric Food Chem* 58:4342–4352 (2010).

[16] Hasnaoui N, Marsa M, Ghaffarib S, Trific M, Melgarejod P and Hernandez F, Seed and juice characterization of pomegranate fruits grown in Tunisia: comparison between sour and sweet cultivars revealed interesting properties for prospective industrial applications. *Ind Crops Prod* 33:374–381 (2011).

[17] Tezcan F, Gültekin-Özgüven M, Diken T, Özçelik B and Erim FB, Antioxidant activity and total phenolic, organic acid and sugar content in commercial pomegranate juices. *Food Chem* 115:873–877 (2009).

[18] Ozgen M, Durgac C, Serce S and Kaya C, Chemical and antioxidant properties of pomegranate cultivars grown in the Mediterranean region of Turkey. *Food Chem* 111:703–706 (2008).

[19] Kader AA, Flavor quality of fruits and vegetables. *J Sci Food Agric* 88:1863–1868 (2008).

[20] Poyrazolua E, Gökmen V and Artık N, Organic acids and phenolic compounds in pomegranates (Punica granatum L.) grown in Turkey. *J Food Comp Anal* 15:567–575 (2002).

[21] Martínez JJ, Hernández F, Abdelmajid H, Legua P, Martínez R, El Amine A, et al, Physico-chemical characterization of six pomegranate cultivars from Morocco: processing and fresh market aptitudes. *Sci Hortic* 140:100–106 (2012)

[22] Gadže J, Voća S, Čmelik Z, Mustać I, Ercisli S and Radunić M, Physico-chemical characteristics of main pomegranate (Punica granatum L.) cultivars grown in the Dalmatia region of Croatia. *J Appl Bot Food Qual* 85:202–206 (2012).

[23] Vardin H and Fenerciog H, Study on the development of pomegranate juice processing technology: clarification of pomegranate juice. *Nahrung/Food* 47:300–303 (2003).

[24] Vázquez-Araújo L, Chambers E, Adhikaria K and Carbonell-Barrachina AA, Physico-chemical and sensory properties of pomegranate juices with pomegranate albedo and carpellar membranes homogenate. *LWT—Food Sci Technol* 44:2119–2125 (2011).

[25] Ben-Arie R, Segal N and Guelfat-Reich S, The maturation and ripening of the 'Wonderful' pomegranate. *J Am Soc Hortic Sci* 109:898–902 (1984).

[26] Al-Maiman, SA and Ahmad D, Changes in physical and chemical properties during pomegranate (Punica granatum L.) fruit maturation. *Food Chem* 76:437–441 (2002).

[27] Kulkarni AP and Aradhya SM, Chemical changes and antioxidant activity in pomegranate arils during fruit development. *Food Chem* 93:319–324 (1995).

[28] Zarei M, Azizi M and Bashir-Sadr Z, Evaluation of physicochemical characteristics of pomegranate (Punica granatum L.) fruit during ripening. *Fruits* 66:121–127 (2009).

[29] Kader AA, Postharvest biology and technology of pomegranates, in *Pomegranates Ancient Roots to Modern Medicine*, ed. by Seeram NP, Schulman RN, Heber D. Taylor & Francis, Boca Raton, FL, pp. 211–220 (2006).

[30] Schwartz E, Tzulker R, Glazer I, Bar-Ya'akov I, Wlesman Z, Tripler E, et al, Environmental conditions affect the color, taste, and antioxidant capacity of 11 pomegranate accessions' fruits. *J Agric Food Chem* 57:9197–9209 (2009).

[31] Zaouay Y, Mena P, Garcia-Viguera C and Mars M, Antioxidant activity and physico-chemical properties of Tunisian grown pomegranate (Punica granatum L.) cultivars. *Ind Crops Prod* 40:81–89 (2012).

[32] Pande G and Akoh CC, Antioxidant capacity and lipid characterization of six Georgia-grown pomegranate cultivars. *J Agric Food Chem* 57:9427–9436 (2009).

[33] Calín-Sánchez A, Martínez JJ, Vázquez-Araújo L, Burló F, Melgarejo P and Carbonell-Barrachina AA, Volatile composition and sensory quality of Spanish pomegranates (Punica granatum L.). *J Sci Food Agric* 91:586–992 (2011).

[34] Melgarejo P, Ín-Sánchez AC, Vázquez-Araújo L, Hernández F, José Martínez J, Legua P and Carbonell-Barrachina AA, Volatile composition of pomegranates from 9 Spanish cultivars using headspace solid phase microextraction. *J Food Sci* 76:114–120 (2011).

[35] Vázquez-Araújo L, Chambers E, Adhikaria K and Carbonell-Barrachina AA, Sensory and physicochemical characterization of juices made with pomegranate and blueberries, blackberries, or raspberries. *J Food Sci* 75:398–404 (2010).

[36] Vázquez-Araújo L, Koppel K, Chambers E, Adhikaria K and Carbonell-Barrachina AA, Instrumental and sensory aroma profile of pomegranate juices from the USA: differences between fresh and commercial juice. *Flav Fragr J* 26:129–138 (2011).

[37] Mayuoni-Kirshinbaum L, Tietel Z, Porat R and Ulrich D, Identification of aroma-active compounds in 'Wonderful' pomegranate fruit using solvent-assisted flavour evaporation and headspace solid-phase micro-extraction methods. *Eur Food Res Technol* 235:277–283 (2012).

[38] Mayuoni-Kirshinbaum L, Daus A and Porat R, Changes in sensory quality and aroma volatile composition during prolonged storage of 'Wonderful' pomegranate fruit. *Int J Food Sci Technol* 48:1569–1578 (2013).

[39] Bajec MR and Pickering GJ, Astringency: mechanisms and perception. *Crit Rev Food Sci Nutr* 48:858–875 (2008).

[40] Fischer UA, Carle R and Kammerer DR, Identification and quantification of phenolic compounds from pomegranate (Punica granatum L.) peel, mesocarp, aril and differently produced juices by HPLC-DAD–ESI/MS. *Food Chem* 127:807–821 (2011).

[41] Qu W, Breska AP, Pan Z and Ma H, Quantitative determination of major polyphenol constituents in pomegranate products. *Food Chem* 132:1585–1591 (2012).

[42] Seeram N, Lee R, Hardy M and Heber D, Rapid large scale purification of ellagitannins from pomegranate husk, a by product of the commercial juice industry. *Sep Purif Technol* 41:49–55 (2005).

[43] Jalikop SH and Kumar PS, Use of soft-, semi-soft- and hard-seeded types of pomegranate (Punica granatum) for improvement of fruit attributes. *Indian J Agric Sci* 68:87–91 (1998).

[44] Martínez JJ, Melgarejo P, Hernández F, Salazar DM and Martínez R, Seed characterization of five new pomegranate (Punica granatum L.) varieties. *Sci Hortic* 110:241–246 (2006).

[45] Sarkhosh A, Zamini Z, Fatahi R and Ranjbar H, Evaluation of genetic diversity among Iranian soft-seed pomegranate accessions by fruit characteristics and RAPD markers. *Sci Hortic* 121:313–319 (2009).

[46] Atres F, Villaaescusa R and Tudela JA, Modified atmosphere packaging of pomegranate. *J Food Sci* 65:1112–1116 (2000).

[47] Porat R, Weiss B, Kosto I, Sandman A and Shachnai A, Modified atmosphere/modified humidity packaging for preserving pomegranate fruit during prolonged storage and transport. *Acta Hortic* 818:299–304 (2009).

Chapter 4

PHARMACOLOGY OF POMEGRANATES

ABSTRACT

Pomegranates have gained significance as a functional food and nutraceutical. The health benefits of pomegranates have been extensively studied. Pomegranates have been shown to be protective against cardiovascular disease, diabetes, neurodegenerative diseases, and a variety of cancers. The *in vitro* antioxidant activity of pomegranate is related to its high polyphenolic content, specifically punicalagins, punicalins, gallagic acid, and ellagic acid. These compounds are metabolized to ellagic acid and urolithins during digestion. It is likely that these bioactive compounds are responsible for the beneficial effects of pomegranates. A complete characterization of pomegranate constituents is necessary to gain a greater understanding of the mechanism of action of potential health benefits due to pomegranate consumption which are observed in clinical trials.

INTRODUCTION

Pomegranates have been consumed as fruits, juices and extracts and used as a medicinal food in the Middle East for thousands of years. Recently, these foods have gained popularity in the developed world due to the potential beneficial effects and strong anti-oxidant properties. The beneficial properties of pomegranate as listed on a number of websites selling pomegranate products to the consumer include its use as an antioxidant, an anti-inflammatory and antiatherogenic treatment. Pomegranate-derived products have been advertised as exhibiting anti-cancer properties, improvement in cardiovascular health, diabetes prevention and management, relief of menopausal symptoms, hormone balance, increased libido in both genders, improved male virility and erectile function, skin nourishment including ant wrinkle effects, and protection against Alzheimer's disease and rheumatoid arthritis. Pomegranates present with far greater high antioxidant activity compared to other fruits and antioxidant beverages [1-10]. This has stimulated interest in research on potential nutraceutical and functional food applications. Unfortunately, the number of popular press, pomegranate-promoting publications far outweighs the number of significantly supportive scientific studies, as evidenced by the approximately 5,700:1 ratio of internet Google™ hits for "pomegranate health" (2,240,000) as compared with a MEDLINE® search for peer-reviewed journal articles on pomegranate. Nonetheless, research on the health benefits of pomegranate has advanced rapidly. The number of peer-reviewed journal articles has nearly doubled in the last two years, and several human clinical trials are currently in progress. Results from these human studies may provide renewed insight on the putative health effects of pomegranate.

Functional Foods and Nutraceutical Products

Apart from its availability as fresh pomegranate fruit, a number of pomegranate-containing products are currently available and advertised with numerous health benefits. These products include 100% juices, pomegranate-containing beverages, liquid and powdered polyphenolic extracts of pomegranate plant parts such as leaves, flowers, arils, and peel, pomegranate seed oil, and skin care products containing pomegranate extracts and/or pomegranate seed oil as ingredients. The rapid growth in demand for pomegranate-based products can be observed by a significant increase in sales of these products from $84,507 in 2001 to $66 million in 2005 in the United States [11].

In respite of this, there is a growing need to standardize the composition of currently available commercial pomegranate juices. One study tested the authenticity of commercially available pomegranate juices from 23 manufacturers based on anthocyanin composition, the presence of pomegranate-specific ellagitannins, sugar, organic acid and amino acid profiles, and potassium content. Of these, only 6 of met the proposed requirements for authenticity. This suggests that several brands of juices are being supplemented with other ingredients or diluted [12]. Similarly, 27 commercially available pomegranate extracts were analyzed for ellagitannin content and in vitro antioxidant capacity. Only 5 contained pomegranate-specific ellagitannins, the punicalins and punicalagins, at significant concentrations. 16 commercial extracts contained primarily ellagic acid, the currently used standardization compound, and five extracts had very little ellagitannin or ellagic acid content and also exhibited low to no antioxidant activity [12]. Punicalagins were only found in extracts that were labeled as such, suggesting that some companies are taking extra measures to produce standardized pomegranate extracts. A major problem in the rapidly growing nutraceutical market is the inverse relationship between production and sales of pomegranate products, and knowledge and standardization. However, continued research on the core bioactive components of pomegranates may hold promise for future products that can correctly deliver the advertised health benefits [13-25].

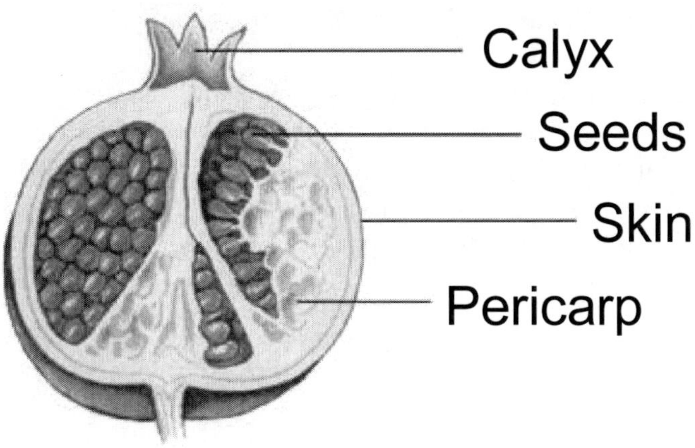

Figure 1. Diagram of pomegranate fruit.

Biochemistry

Multiple antioxidant activity assays have shown that pomegranate fruit and juices have demonstrated antioxidant properties greater than other foods considered to have high antioxidant activity, including red wine and green tea [26-45]. The major bioactive phytochemical compounds present in pomegranates include anthocyanins and hydrolyzable tannins, specifically ellagitannins, which release ellagic acid when hydrolyzed. Punicalagin, punicalin, gallagic acid, and ellagic acid were found to account for the majority of the ellagitannins in pomegranate juices and homogenates from 29 lines over two growing seasons [46]. The strong antioxidant activity of pomegranate juices as measured by trolox equivalent antioxidant capacity (TEAC) and ascorbic acid equivalent antioxidant capacity (AEAC) is due to the concentration of these hydrolyzable tannins, with anthocyanins contributing very little to in vitro antioxidant capacity [47]. In whole fruit pomegranate homogenates, antioxidant activity was also correlated significantly with total polyphenols ($R^2 = 0.90$, $P < 0.01$), but not with total anthocyanin content ($R^2 = 0.05$, $P > 0.05$) [48]. Nevertheless, anthocyanins have been associated with health effects, including prevention of cardiovascular disease, obesity, and diabetes [49] and should not be ignored as potentially bioactive components of pomegranate. The major anthocyanins in pomegranate juice are delphinidin 3,5-diglucoside, cyanidin 3,5-diglucoside, pelargonidin 3,5-diglucoside, delphinidin 3-glucoside, cyanidin 3-glucoside, and pelargonidin 3-glucoside [50].

Pomegranate peel extracts have a greater antioxidant activity than the juice or seed extracts. They have been shown to prevent the formation of lipid peroxidation and low-density lipoprotein (LDL) oxidation. Additionally, pomegranate peel extract showed greater antioxidant capabilities than turmeric or ascorbic acid (vitamin C), two well-known antioxidants [51-55].

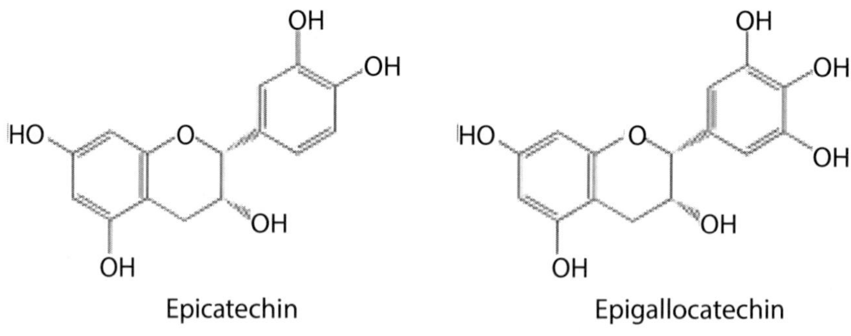

Figure 2. Main catechins found in pomegranates.

Pomegranate seeds have a lower polyphenol content and in vitro antioxidant capacity [56]. However, the seed oil is rich in phytosterols and a unique fatty acid profile that includes punicic acid, a conjugated linolenic acid isomer [57]. Punicic acid concentrations constitute 70% to 76% of the pomegranate seed oil. Other constituents of pomegranate oils include α-eleostearic, linoleic, oleic, catalpic, palmitic, stearic, β-eleostearic, gadoleic, arachidic, and behenic acids [58].

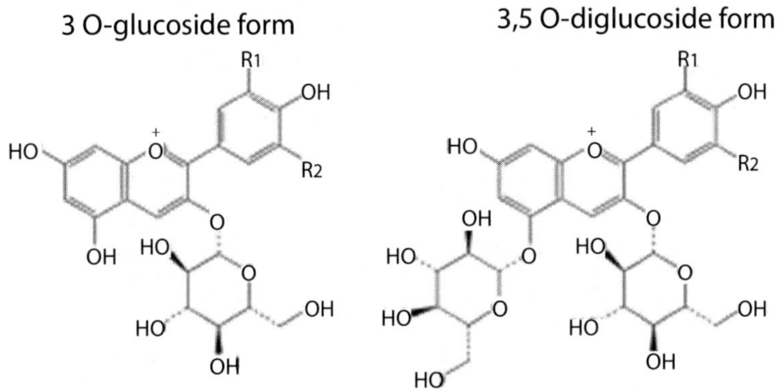

Figure 3. Main anthrocyanins, as 3-O[glucoside and 3,5-O-glucoside forms found in pomegranates.

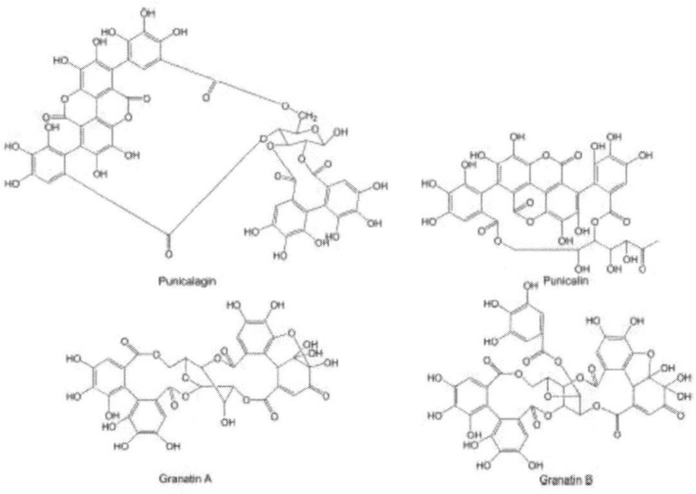

Figure 4. Punicalgins and granatins found in pomegranates.

Table 1. Constituents of pomegranates

Compound class	Compounds	
Diverse polyphenols[29-33]	Catechin	Gallocatechin
	Ellagic acid	Kaempferol
	Epicatechin	Luteolin
	Epigallocatechin	Quercetin
Ellagitannins[29,30,31,34-38]	Brevifolin	Lagerstannin B
	Brevifolin carboxylic acid	Pedunculagin
	Corilagin	Pomegranatate
	Castalagin	Punicafolin
	Casuarinin	Punicalin
	Gallagyldilactone	Punicalagin A
	Granatin A	Punicalagin B
	Granatin B	Tellimagrandin I
Anthocyanins[29,30,32,39-42]	Pelargonidin 3 *O*-glucoside	Cyanidin 3,5 O-diglucoside
	Pelargonidin 3,5 *O*-diglucoside	Delphinidin 3 O-glucoside
	Cyanidin 3 *O*-glucoside	Delphinidin 3,5 O-diglucoside
Volatile compounds[43-47]	*E*-α-Bergamotene	*trans*-2-Hexenal
	E-β-Bergamotene	*cis*-3-Hexenol
	Bisabolene	Heptanal
	Cadrene	Limonene
	Camphor	Menthol
	3-Carene	β-Myrcene
	β-Caryophyllene	Nonanal
	p-Cumic aldehyde	Octanal
	p-Cymene	α-Phellandrene
	(*Z*,*Z*)-α-Farnesene	α-Pinene
	β-Farnesene	β-Pinene
	Fenchone	α-Terpinene
	Furfural	γ-Terpinene
	Hexanal	4-Terpineol
	Hexanol	α-Terpineol
	cis-3-Hexenal	
Organic & phenolic acids[29,44-50]	Ascorbic acid	Gallic acid
	Caffeic acid	Malic acid
	Chlorogenic acid	Oxalic acid
	Citric acid	(-)-Quinic acid
	o-Coumaric acid	Succinic acid
	p-Coumaric acid	Tartaric acid
	Ferulic acid	
Fatty acids[51-57]	Caproic acid ($C_{6:0}$)	Linoleic acid ($C_{18:2}$)
	Caprylic acid ($C_{8:0}$)	Punicic acid ($C_{18:3}$, 9-cis, 11-*trans*, 13-*cis*)
	Capric acid ($C_{10:0}$)	α-Eleostearic acid ($C_{18:3}$, 9-cis, 11-*trans*, 13-*trans*)
	Lauric acid ($C_{12:0}$)	β-Eleostearic acid ($C_{18:3}$, 9-*trans*, 11-*trans*, 13-*trans*)
	Myristic acid ($C_{14:0}$)	Catalpic acid ($C_{18:3}$, 9-*trans*, 11-*trans*, 13-*cis*)
	Myristoleic acid ($C_{14:1}$)	Arachidic acid ($C_{20:0}$)
	Palmitic acid ($C_{16:0}$)	Gadoleic acid ($C_{20:1}$)
	Palmitoleic acid ($C_{16:1}$)	Lignoceric acid ($C_{24:0}$)
	Stearic acid ($C_{18:0}$)	Nervonic acid ($C_{24:1}$, 15-*cis*)
	Oleic acid ($C_{18:1}$)	
Lignans[58]	Isolariciresinol	Pinoresinol
	Matairesinol (only in wood knots)	Secoisolariciresinol
	Medioresinol	Syringaresinol

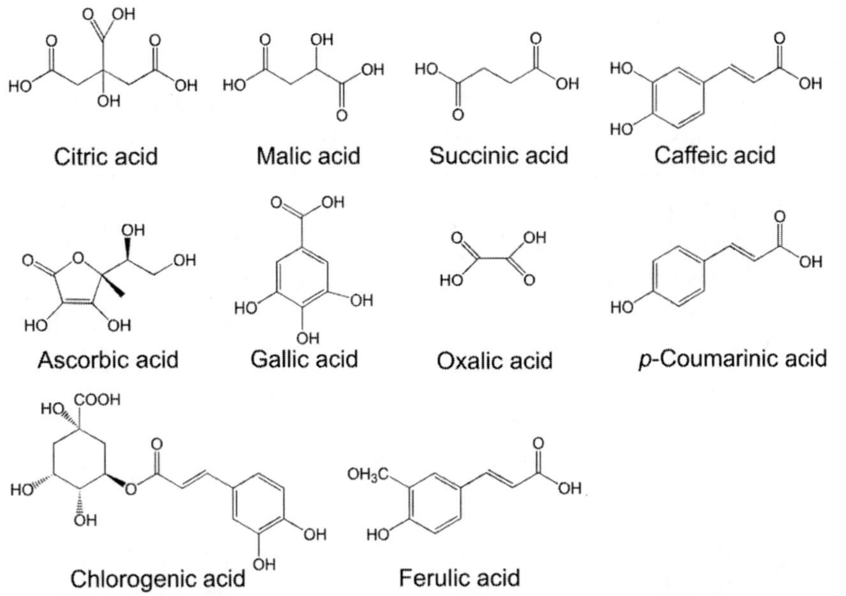

Figure 5. Phenolic acids present in pomegranates.

BIOAVAILABILITY

The high in vitro antioxidant capacity of pomegranate products is largely due to the high content of polyphenolic compounds, particularly ellagitannins. In studies of ellagitannin bioavailability in human subjects, ellagic acid and its metabolites were detected in the plasma of individual's post-pomegranate juice consumption [59-65]. No difference in bioavailability has been reported for pomegranate juice, liquid extract, or powdered extract forms of treatment as measured by plasma ellagic acid or its metabolites that contained similar levels of total polyphenols standardized as gallic acid equivalents [66-70].

On the contrary, another study showed that no ellagic acid, punicalagin, anthocyanins, or their biological degradation products are present in plasma after pomegranate juice consumption (1 litre per day distributed in 5–200 mL bottles), despite high levels of ellagic acid and punicalagin in the juices. Interestingly, the study identified urolithin metabolites which were indicative of extensive colonic microbial metabolism of the pomegranate juice polyphenols [71]. The apparent discrepancies between the two studies may be due to significant variation between the timing of plasma samples, and the short half-life of ellagic acid in the plasma [72].

Using acorn-fed Iberian pigs as a model system, 31 ellagitannin metabolites were detected. However, only urolithin A, urolithin B, dimethyl ellagic acid and their glucuronide derivatives were found in plasma [73]. Urolithin metabolites have been shown to be readily absorbed in mouse models, with the highest levels accumulated in prostate, colon, and intestinal tissues [74]. Similarly, urolithin A glucuronide, urolithin B glucuronide, and dimethylellagic acid were the only ellagic acid metabolites detected in human prostate tissues after three days of supplementation with pomegranate juice [75]. It is likely that ellagitannins are hydrolyzed in the stomach where some portion of ellagic acid may be absorbed into circulation. The remaining ellagic acid is metabolized to urolithin derivatives by gut microflora. The less polar of these urolithin derivatives (A and B) are absorbed into circulation and metabolized further to glucuronides [76-80].

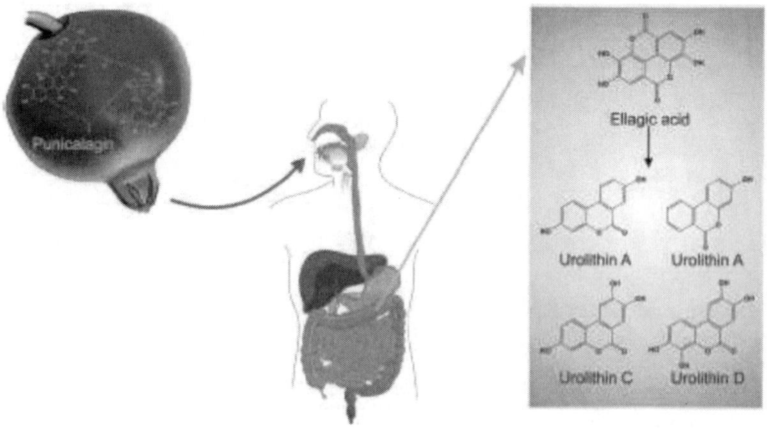

Figure 6. Catabolism of Punicalgins.

Toxicity and Potential Drug Interactions

It is generally considered safe to consume the fresh fruit and juice of pomegranates, and no adverse effects have reported in human clinical trials. Toxicity studies have been carried out in rat and mouse models. The lethal dose 50 (LD50) for pomegranate fruit extract standardized to 30% punicalagins was found to be greater than 5 g kg^{-1} body weight [81-85]. In another toxicological study, rat diets were replaced with a 20% pomegranate powder:80% rat chow diet that resulted in 6% punicalagin (equilibrated concentration). This diet was fed for 37 days with no evidence of toxicity [86]. Similarly, no significant negative effects or changes in renal or liver function parameters in a study of 64 overweight individuals given POMx brand pomegranate extract powder (1 or 2 capsules daily versus placebo) over the course of a 28 day treatment period [86]. As well, no observable adverse effect level was reported for pomegranate seed oil [87].

Research in rat models has shown that pomegranate juice inhibited cytochrome P450 enzymes CYP2C9 [88] and CYP3A [89] in vitro and increased levels of absorbed tolbutamide and carbamazepine by increasing bioavailability. However, no effect on the clearance of these compounds by the corresponding liver enzymes [90] has been reported. Consumption of pomegranate juice for four weeks in a mouse model showed an overall decrease in liver CYP450 concentration and an increase in the sleep effect induced by pentobarbital. The decrease in total CYP450 was attributed to decreases in liver CYP1A2 and 3A. Although pomegranate juice inhibited CYP3A in vitro, there was no effect on midazolam metabolism post-pomegranate juice consumption [91]. Further research is needed to fully understand the interaction of pomegranate products with CYP450 enzymes and the implications of those interactions for human health [92-95].

Future Directions and Conclusion

Recent human clinical trials have shown significant positive effects of pomegranate juice consumption on lipid profiles in diabetic patients, atherosclerosis reduction and on PSA levels in prostate cancer patients. Although these human studies are limited in number, they show evidence that regular consumption of pomegranate juice may aid in the prevention or management of chronic diseases. A more complete characterization of the bioactive components of pomegranate products and their physiological actions will be required to study the underlying mechanisms for the potential health benefits that have been demonstrated in clinical trials.

References

[1] Adams, L. S., Seeram, N. P., Aggarwal, B. B., Takada, Y., Sand, D. and Heber, D. 2006. Pomegranate juice, total pomegranate ellagitannins, and punicalagin suppress inflammatory cell signaling in colon cancer cells. *J Agric Food Chem*, 54(3): 980–985.

[2] Afaq, F., Malik, A., Syed, D., Maes, D., Matsui, M. S. and Mukhtar, H. 2005. Pomegranate fruit extract modulates UV-B-mediated phosphorylation of mitogen-activated protein kinases and activation of nuclear factor kappa B in normal human epidermal keratinocytes paragraph sign. *Photochem Photobiol*, 81(1): 38–45.

[3] Albrecht, M., Jiang, W., Kumi-Diaka, J., Lansky, E. P., Gommersall, L. M., Patel, A., Mansel, R. E., Neeman, I., Geldof, A. A. and Campbell, M. J. 2004. Pomegranate extracts potently suppress proliferation, xenograft growth, and invasion of human prostate cancer cells. *J Med Food*, 7(3): 274–283.

[4] Alper, N., Bahceci, K. S. and Acar, J. 2005. Influence of processing and pasteurization on color values and total phenolic compounds of pomegranate juice. *J. Food Process Preserv*, 29(5–6): 357–368.

[5] Aslam, M. N., Lansky, E. P. and Varani, J. 2006. Pomegranate as a cosmeceutical source: pomegranate fractions promote proliferation and procollagen synthesis and inhibit matrix metalloproteinase-1 production in human skin cells. *J Ethnopharmacol*, 103(3): 311–318.

[6] Aviram, M. and Dornfeld, L. 2001. Pomegranate juice consumption inhibits serum angiotensin converting enzyme activity and reduces systolic blood pressure. *Atherosclerosis*, 158(1): 195–198.

[7] Aviram, M., Dornfeld, L., Rosenblat, M., Volkova, N., Kaplan, M., Coleman, R., Hayek, T., Presser, D. and Fuhrman, B. 2000. Pomegranate juice consumption reduces oxidative stress, atherogenic modifications to LDL, and platelet aggregation: Studies in humans and in atherosclerotic apolipoprotein E-deficient mice. *Am J Clin Nutr*, 71(5): 1062–1076.

[8] Aviram, M., Rosenblat, M., Gaitini, D., Nitecki, S., Hoffman, A., Dornfeld, L., Volkova, N., Presser, D., Attias, J., Liker, H. and Hayek, T. 2004. Pomegranate juice consumption for 3 years by patients with carotid artery stenosis reduces common carotid intima-media thickness, blood pressure and LDL oxidation. *Clin Nutr*, 23(3): 423–433.

[9] Aviram, M., Volkova, N., Coleman, R., Dreher, M., Reddy, M. K., Ferreira, D. and Rosenblat, M. 2008. Pomegranate phenolics from the

peels, arils, and flowers are antiatherogenic: Studies in vivo in atherosclerotic apolipoprotein e-deficient (E 0) mice and in vitro in cultured macrophages and lipoproteins. *J Agric Food Chem*, 56(3): 1148–1157.

[10] Benzie, I. F. 2003. Evolution of dietary antioxidants. *Comp Biochem Physiol A Mol Integr Physiol*, 136(1): 113–126.

[11] Bialonska, D., Kasimsetty, S. G., Khan, S. I. and Ferreira, D. 2009. Urolithins, intestinal microbial metabolites of Pomegranate ellagitannins, exhibit potent antioxidant activity in a cell-based assay. *J Agric Food Chem*, 57(21): 10181–10186.

[12] Caceres, A., Giron, L. M., Alvarado, S. R. and Torres, M. F. 1987. Screening of antimicrobial activity of plants popularly used in Guatemala for the treatment of dermatomucosal diseases. *J Ethnopharmacol*, 20(3): 223–237.

[13] Cerda, B., Ceron, J. J., Tomas-Barberan, F. A. and Espin, J. C. 2003. Repeated oral administration of high doses of the pomegranate ellagitannin punicalagin to rats for 37 days is not toxic. *J Agric Food Chem*, 51(11): 3493–3501.

[14] Cerda, B., Periago, P., Espin, J. C. and Tomas-Barberan, F. A. 2005. Identification of urolithin A as a metabolite produced by human colon microflora from ellagic acid and related compounds. *J. Agric. Food Chem*, 53(14): 5571–5576.

[15] Chidambara Murthy, K. N., Jayaprakasha, G. K. and Singh, R. P. 2002. Studies on antioxidant activity of pomegranate (Punica granatum) peel extract using in vivo models. *J Agric Food Chem*, 50(17): 4791–4795.

[16] Conner, E. M. and Grisham, M. B. 1996. Inflammation, free radicals, and antioxidants. *Nutrition*, 12(4): 274–277.

[17] Curry, S. C. 2004. “Breast enhancement system”. US pat. 6673366.

[18] de Nigris, F, Balestrieri, M. L., Williams-Ignarro, S., D’Armiento, F. P., Fiorito, C., Ignarro, L. J. and Napoli, C. 2007. The influence of pomegranate fruit extract in comparison to regular pomegranate juice and seed oil on nitric oxide and arterial function in obese Zucker rats. *Nitric Oxide*, 17(1): 50–54.

[19] Faria, A., Monteiro, R., Azevedo, I. and Calhau, C. 2007a. Pomegranate juice effects on cytochrome P450S expression: In vivo studies. *J Med Food*, 10(4): 643–649.

[20] Faria, A., Monteiro, R., Mateus, N., Azevedo, I. and Calhau, C. 2007b. Effect of pomegranate (Punica granatum) juice intake on hepatic oxidative stress. *Eur. J. Nutr*, 46(5): 271–278.

[21] Farkas, D., Oleson, L. E., Zhao, Y., Harmatz, J. S., Zinny, M. A., Court, M. H. and Greenblatt, D. J. 2007. Pomegranate juice does not impair clearance of oral or intravenous midazolam, a probe for cytochrome P450–3A activity: Comparison with grapefruit juice. *J Clin Pharmacol*, 47(3): 286–294.

[22] Gil, M. I., Tomas-Barberan, F. A., Hess-Pierce, B., Holcroft, D. M. and Kader, A. A. 2000. Antioxidant activity of pomegranate juice and its relationship with phenolic composition and processing. *J Agric Food Chem*, 48(10): 4581–4589.

[23] Guo, C. J., Yang, J. J., Wei, J. Y., Li, Y. F., Xu, J. and Jiang, Y. G. 2003. Antioxidant activities of peel, pulp and seed fractions of common fruits as determined by FRAP assay. *Nutr. Res*, 23(12): 1719–1726.

[24] Guo, S., Deng, Q., Xiao, J., Xie, B. and Sun, Z. 2007. Evaluation of antioxidant activity and preventing DNA damage effect of pomegranate extracts by chemiluminescence method. *J Agric Food Chem*, 55(8): 3134–3140.

[25] Hajimahmoodi, M., Oveisi, M. R., Sadeghi, N., Jannat, B., Hadjibabaie, M., Farahani, E., Akrami, M. R. and Namdar, R. 2008. Antioxidant properties of peel and pulp hydro extract in ten Persian pomegranate cultivars. *Pak J Biol Sci*, 11(12): 1600–1604.

[26] Heber, D. 2008. Multitargeted therapy of cancer by ellagitannins. *Cancer Lett*, 269(2): 262–268.

[27] Heber, D., Seeram, N. P., Wyatt, H., Henning, S. M., Zhang, Y., Ogden, L. G., Dreher, M. and Hill, J. O. 2007. Safety and antioxidant activity of a pomegranate ellagitannin-enriched polyphenol dietary supplement in overweight individuals with increased waist size. *J Agric Food Chem*, 55(24): 10050–10054.

[28] Heim, K. E., Tagliaferro, A. R. and Bobilya, D. J. 2002. Flavonoid antioxidants: chemistry, metabolism and structure-activity relationships. *J Nutr Biochem*, 13(10): 572–584.

[29] Hidaka, M., Fujita, K., Ogikubo, T., Yamasaki, K., Iwakiri, T., Okumura, M., Kodama, H. and Arimori, K. 2004. Potent inhibition by star fruit of human cytochrome P450 3A (CYP3A) activity. *Drug Metab Dispos*, 32(6): 581–583.

[30] Hidaka, M., Okumura, M., Fujita, K., Ogikubo, T., Yamasaki, K., Iwakiri, T., Setoguchi, N. and Arimori, K. 2005. Effects of pomegranate juice on human cytochrome p450 3A (CYP3A) and carbamazepine pharmacokinetics in rats. *Drug Metab Dispos*, 33(5): 644–648.

[31] Hontecillas, R., O'Shea, M., Einerhand, A., Diguardo, M. and Bassaganya-Riera, J. 2009. Activation of PPAR gamma and alpha by punicic acid ameliorates glucose tolerance and suppresses obesity-related inflammation. *J Am Coll Nutr*, 28(2): 184–195.

[32] Hora, J. J., Maydew, E. R., Lansky, E. P. and Dwivedi, C. 2003. Chemopreventive effects of pomegranate seed oil on skin tumor development in CD1 mice. *Journal of Medicinal Food*, 6(3): 157–161.

[33] Huang, T. H., Peng, G., Kota, B. P., Li, G. Q., Yamahara, J., Roufogalis, B. D. and Li, Y. 2005. Pomegranate flower improves cardiac lipid metabolism in a diabetic rat model: Role of lowering circulating lipids. *Br J Pharmacol*, 145(6): 767–774.

[34] Kaplan, M., Hayek, T., Raz, A., Coleman, R., Dornfeld, L., Vaya, J. and Aviram, M. 2001. Pomegranate juice supplementation to atherosclerotic mice reduces macrophage lipid peroxidation, cellular cholesterol accumulation and development of atherosclerosis. *J Nutr*, 131(8): 2082–2089.

[35] Kaufman, M. and Wiesman, Z. 2007. Pomegranate oil analysis with emphasis on MALDI-TOF/MS triacylglycerol fingerprinting. *J Agric Food Chem*, 55(25): 10405–10413.

[36] Kaur, G., Jabbar, Z., Athar, M. and Alam, M. S. 2006. Punica granatum (pomegranate) flower extract possesses potent antioxidant activity and abrogates Fe-NTA induced hepatotoxicity in mice. *Food Chem Toxicol*, 44(7): 984–993.

[37] Kehrer, J. P. 1993. Free radicals as mediators of tissue injury and disease. *Crit Rev Toxicol*, 23(1): 21–48.

[38] Khan, G. N., Gorin, M. A., Rosenthal, D., Pan, Q., Bao, L. W., Wu, Z. F., Newman, R. A., Pawlus, A. D., Yang, P., Lansky, E. P. and Merajver, S. D. 2009. Pomegranate fruit extract impairs invasion and motility in human breast cancer. *Integr Cancer Ther*, 8(3): 242–253.

[39] Kim, H., Yoon, Y. J., Shon, J. H., Cha, I. J., Shin, J. G. and Liu, K. H. 2006. Inhibitory effects of fruit juices on CYP3A activity. *Drug Metab Dispos*, 34(4): 521–523.

[40] Kim, N. D., Mehta, R., Yu, W., Neeman, I., Livney, T., Amichay, A., Poirier, D., Nicholls, P., Kirby, A., Jiang, W., Mansel, R., Ramachandran, C., Rabi, T., Kaplan, B. and Lansky, E. 2002. Chemopreventive and adjuvant therapeutic potential of pomegranate (Punica granatum) for human breast cancer. *Breast Cancer Res Treat*, 71(3): 203–217.

[41] Kohno, H., Suzuki, R., Yasui, Y., Hosokawa, M., Miyashita, K. and Tanaka, T. 2004. Pomegranate seed oil rich in conjugated linolenic acid suppresses chemically induced colon carcinogenesis in rats. *Cancer Sci*, 95(6): 481–486.

[42] Kulkarni, A. P., Mahal, H. S., Kapoor, S. and Aradhya, S. M. 2007. In vitro studies on the binding, antioxidant, and cytotoxic actions of punicalagin. *J Agric Food Chem*, 55(4): 1491–1500.

[43] Lansky, E. P. and Newman, R. A. 2007. Punica granatum (pomegranate) and its potential for prevention and treatment of inflammation and cancer. *J Ethnopharmacol*, 109(2): 177–206.

[44] Larrosa, M., Gonzalez-Sarrias, A., Yanez-Gascon, M. J., Selma, M. V., Azorin-Ortuno, M., Toti, S., Tomas-Barberan, F., Dolara, P. and Espin, J. C. 2010. Anti-inflammatory properties of a pomegranate extract and its metabolite urolithin-A in a colitis rat model and the effect of colon inflammation on phenolic metabolism. *J Nutr Biochem*, 21(8): 717–725.

[45] Larrosa, M., Tomas-Barberan, F. A. and Espin, J. C. 2006. The dietary hydrolysable tannin punicalagin releases ellagic acid that induces apoptosis in human colon adenocarcinoma Caco-2 cells by using the mitochondrial pathway. *J Nutr Biochem*, 17(9): 611–625.

[46] Lei, F., Zhang, X. N., Wang, W., Xing, D. M., Xie, W. D., Su, H. and Du, L. J. 2007. Evidence of anti-obesity effects of the pomegranate leaf extract in high-fat diet induced obese mice. *Int J Obes (Lond)*, 31(6): 1023–1029.

[47] Li, Y., Qi, Y., Huang, T. H., Yamahara, J. and Roufogalis, B. D. 2008. Pomegranate flower: A unique traditional antidiabetic medicine with dual PPAR-alpha/-gamma activator properties. *Diabetes Obes Metab*, 10(1): 10–17.

[48] Li, Y. F., Guo, C. J., Yang, J. J., Wei, J. Y., Xu, J. and Cheng, S. 2006. Evaluation of antioxidant properties of pomegranate peel extract in comparison with pomegranate pulp extract. *Food Chem*, 96(2): 254–260.

[49] Lin, C. C., Hsu, Y. F. and Lin, T. C. 1999. Effects of punicalagin and punicalin on carrageenan-induced inflammation in rats. *Am J Chin Med*, 27(3–4): 371–376.

[50] Lin, C. C., Hsu, Y. F., Lin, T. C., Hsu, F. L. and Hsu, H. Y. 1998. Antioxidant and hepatoprotective activity of punicalagin and punicalin on carbon tetrachloride-induced liver damage in rats. *J Pharm Pharmacol*, 50(7): 789–794.

[51] Lin, C. C., Hsu, Y. F., Lin, T. C. and Hsu, H. Y. 2001. Antioxidant and hepatoprotective effects of punicalagin and punicalin on acetaminophen-induced liver damage in rats. *Phytother Res*, 15(3): 206–212.

[52] Mahdihassan, S. 1984. Outline of the beginnings of alchemy and its antecedents. *Am J Chin Med*, 12(1–4): 32–42.

[53] Malik, A., Afaq, F., Sarfaraz, S., Adhami, V. M., Syed, D. N. and Mukhtar, H. 2005. Pomegranate fruit juice for chemoprevention and chemotherapy of prostate cancer. *Proc Natl Acad Sci U S A*, 102(41): 14813–14818.

[54] Martin, I. and Grotewiel, M. S. 2006. Oxidative damage and age-related functional declines. *Mech Ageing Dev*, 127(5): 411–423.

[55] Masella, R., Di Benedetto, R., Vari, R., Filesi, C. and Giovannini, C. 2005. Novel mechanisms of natural antioxidant compounds in biological systems: Involvement of glutathione and glutathione-related enzymes. *J Nutr Biochem*, 16(10): 577–586.

[56] Meerts, I. A., Verspeek-Rip, C. M., Buskens, C. A., Keizer, H. G., Bassaganya-Riera, J., Jouni, Z. E., van Huygevoort, A. H., van Otterdijk, F. M. and van de Waart, E. J. 2009. Toxicological evaluation of pomegranate seed oil. *Food Chem Toxicol*, 47(6): 1085–1092.

[57] Mehta, R. and Lansky, E. P. 2004. Breast cancer chemopreventive properties of pomegranate (Punica granatum) fruit extracts in a mouse mammary organ culture. *Eur J Cancer Prev*, 13(4): 345–348.

[58] Mertens-Talcott, S. U., Jilma-Stohlawetz, P., Rios, J., Hingorani, L. and Derendorf, H. 2006. Absorption, metabolism, and antioxidant effects of pomegranate (Punica granatum l.) polyphenols after ingestion of a standardized extract in healthy human volunteers. *J Agric Food Chem*, 54(23): 8956–8961.

[59] Mirdehghan, S. H. and Rahemi, M. 2007. Seasonal changes of mineral nutrients and phenolics in pomegranate (Punica granatum L.) fruit. *Sci. Hortic*, 111(2): 120–127.

[60] Nagata, M., Hidaka, M., Sekiya, H., Kawano, Y., Yamasaki, K., Okumura, M. and Arimori, K. 2007. Effects of pomegranate juice on human cytochrome P450 2C9 and tolbutamide pharmacokinetics in rats. *Drug Metab Dispos*, 35(2): 302–305.

[61] Naqvi, S. A. H., Khan, M. S. Y. and Vohora, S. B. 1991. Anti-bacterial anti-fungal and anthelmintic investigations on indian medicinal plants. *Fitoterapia*, 62(3): 221–228.

[62] Negi, P. S., Jayaprakasha, G. K. and Jena, B. S. 2003. Antioxidant and antimutagenic activities of pomegranate peel extracts. *Food Chem.*, 80(3): 393–397.

[63] Obach, R. S. 2000. Inhibition of human cytochrome P450 enzymes by constituents of St. John's Wort, an herbal preparation used in the treatment of depression. *J Pharmacol Exp Ther*, 294(1): 88–95.

[64] Okamoto, T., Akuta, T., Tamura, F., Van Der Vliet, A. and Akaike, T. 2004. Molecular mechanism for activation and regulation of matrix metalloproteinases during bacterial infections and respiratory inflammation. *Biol Chem*, 385(11): 997–1006.

[65] Okonogi, S., Duangrat, C., Anuchpreeda, S., Tachakittirungrod, S. and Chowwanapoonpohn, S. 2007. Comparison of antioxidant capacities and cytotoxicities of certain fruit peels. *Food Chem*, 103(3): 839–846.

[66] Pastorekova, S., Parkkila, S., Pastorek, J. and Supuran, C. T. 2004. Carbonic anhydrases: current state of the art, therapeutic applications and future prospects. *J Enzyme Inhib Med Chem*, 19(3): 199–229.

[67] Patel, C., Dadhaniya, P., Hingorani, L. and Soni, M. G. 2008. Safety assessment of pomegranate fruit extract: acute and subchronic toxicity studies. *Food Chem Toxicol*, 46(8): 2728–2735.

[68] Patterson, L. H. and Murray, G. I. 2002. Tumour cytochrome P450 and drug activation. *Curr Pharm Des*, 8(15): 1335–1347.

[69] Rasheed, Z., Akhtar, N., Anbazhagan, A. N., Ramamurthy, S., Shukla, M. and Haqqi, T. M. 2009. Polyphenol-rich pomegranate fruit extract (POMx) suppresses PMACI-induced expression of pro-inflammatory cytokines by inhibiting the activation of MAP Kinases and NF-kappaB in human KU812 cells. *J Inflamm (Lond)*, 6: 1–12.

[70] Rice-Evans, C. A., Miller, N. J. and Paganga, G. 1996. Structure-antioxidant activity relationships of flavonoids and phenolic acids. *Free Radic Biol Med*, 20(7): 933–956.

[71] Rosenblat, M., Hayek, T. and Aviram, M. 2006. Anti-oxidative effects of pomegranate juice (PJ) consumption by diabetic patients on serum and on macrophages. *Atherosclerosis*, 187(2): 363–371.

[72] Ross, J. A. and Kasum, C. M. 2002. Dietary flavonoids: bioavailability, metabolic effects, and safety. *Annu Rev Nutr*, 22: 19–34.

[73] Rozenberg, O., Howell, A. and Aviram, M. 2006. Pomegranate juice sugar fraction reduces macrophage oxidative state, whereas white grape juice sugar fraction increases it. *Atherosclerosis*, 188(1): 68–76.

[74] Satomi, H., Umemura, K., Ueno, A., Hatano, T., Okuda, T. and Noro, T. 1993. Carbonic anhydrase inhibitors from the pericarps of Punica granatum L. *Biol Pharm Bull*, 16(8): 787–790.

[75] Schubert, S. Y., Lansky, E. P. and Neeman, I. 1999. Antioxidant and eicosanoid enzyme inhibition properties of pomegranate seed oil and fermented juice flavonoids. *J Ethnopharmacol*, 66(1): 11–17.

[76] Seeram, N. P., Adams, L. S., Henning, S. M., Niu, Y., Zhang, Y., Nair, M. G. and Heber, D. 2005. In vitro antiproliferative, apoptotic and antioxidant activities of punicalagin, ellagic acid and a total pomegranate tannin extract are enhanced in combination with other polyphenols as found in pomegranate juice. *J Nutr Biochem*, 16(6): 360–367.

[77] Seeram, N. P., Aronson, W. J., Zhang, Y., Henning, S. M., Moro, A., Lee, R. P., Sartippour, M., Harris, D. M., Rettig, M., Suchard, M. A., Pantuck, A. J., Belldegrun, A. and Heber, D. 2007a. Pomegranate ellagitannin-derived metabolites inhibit prostate cancer growth and localize to the mouse prostate gland. *J Agric Food Chem*, 55(19): 7732–7737.

[78] Seeram, N. P., Aviram, M., Zhang, Y., Henning, S. M., Feng, L., Dreher, M. and Heber, D. 2008. Comparison of antioxidant potency of commonly consumed polyphenol-rich beverages in the United States. *J Agric Food Chem*, 56(4): 1415–1422.

[79] Seeram, N. P., Henning, S. M., Zhang, Y., Suchard, M., Li, Z. and Heber, D. 2006. Pomegranate juice ellagitannin metabolites are present in human plasma and some persist in urine for up to 48 hours. *J Nutr*, 136(10): 2481–2485.

[80] Seeram, N. P., Zhang, Y. J., Sartipipour, M., Henning, S. M., Lee, R. P., Harris, D. M., Moro, A. and Heber, D. 2007b. "Pharmacokinetics and tissue disposition of urolithin A, an ellagitannin-derived metabolite, in mice". In *Experimental Biology 2007 Annual Meeting*, A1081–A1081. Washington, DC: Federation Amer Soc Exp Biol.

[81] Shukla, M., Gupta, K., Rasheed, Z., Khan, K. A. and Haqqi, T. M. 2008. Bioavailable constituents/metabolites of pomegranate (Punica granatum L) preferentially inhibit COX2 activity ex vivo and IL-1beta-induced PGE2 production in human chondrocytes in vitro. *J Inflamm (Lond)*, 5: 9–19.

[82] Shukla, S. and Gupta, S. 2004. Molecular mechanisms for apigenin-induced cell-cycle arrest and apoptosis of hormone refractory human prostate carcinoma DU145 cells. *Mol Carcinog*, 39(2): 114–126.

[83] Singh, R. P., Chidambara Murthy, K. N. and Jayaprakasha, G. K. 2002. Studies on the antioxidant activity of pomegranate (Punica granatum) peel and seed extracts using in vitro models. *J Agric Food Chem*, 50(1): 81–86.

[84] Sparreboom, A., Cox, M. C., Acharya, M. R. and Figg, W. D. 2004. Herbal remedies in the United States: Potential adverse interactions with anticancer agents. *J Clin Oncol*, 22(12): 2489–2503.

[85] Storz, P. 2005. Reactive oxygen species in tumor progression. *Front Biosci*, 10: 1881–1896.

[86] Syed, D. N., Afaq, F. and Mukhtar, H. 2007. Pomegranate derived products for cancer chemoprevention. *Semin Cancer Biol*, 17(5): 377–385.

[87] Tapiero, H., Tew, K. D., Ba, G. N. and Mathe, G. 2002. Polyphenols: Do they play a role in the prevention of human pathologies?. *Biomed Pharmacother*, 56(4): 200–207.

[88] Terman, A. and Brunk, U. T. 2006. Oxidative stress, accumulation of biological "garbage" and aging. *Antioxid Redox Signal*, 8: 1–2. 197–204.

[89] Toi, M., Bando, H., Ramachandran, C., Melnick, S. J., Imai, A., Fife, R. S., Carr, R. E., Oikawa, T. and Lansky, E. P. 2003. Preliminary studies on the anti-angiogenic potential of pomegranate fractions in vitro and in vivo. *Angiogenesis*, 6(2): 121–128.

[90] Toklu, H. Z., Dumlu, M. U., Sehirli, O., Ercan, F., Gedik, N., Gokmen, V. and Sener, G. 2007. Pomegranate peel extract prevents liver fibrosis in biliary-obstructed rats. *J Pharm Pharmacol*, 59(9): 1287–1295.

[91] Tsuyuki, H., Itoh, S. and Nakatsukasa, Y. 1981. Studies on the lipids in pomegranate punica-granatum-var-nana seeds. *Bulletin of the College of Agriculture and Veterinary Medicine Nihon University*, : 141–148.

[92] Wang, Z., Gorski, J. C., Hamman, M. A., Huang, S. M., Lesko, L. J. and Hall, S. D. 2001. The effects of St John's wort (Hypericum perforatum) on human cytochrome P450 activity. *Clin Pharmacol Ther*, 70(4): 317–326.

[93] Williams, R. J., Spencer, J. P. and Rice-Evans, C. 2004. Flavonoids: Antioxidants or signalling molecules?. *Free Radic Biol Med*, 36(7): 838–849.

[94] Yamasaki, M., Kitagawa, T., Koyanagi, N., Chujo, H., Maeda, H., Kohno-Murase, J., Imamura, J., Tachibana, H. and Yamada, K. 2006. Dietary effect of pomegranate seed oil on immune function and lipid metabolism in mice. *Nutrition*, 22(1): 54–59.

[95] Zhu, Y. S., Cai, L. Q., Huang, Y., Fish, J., Wang, L., Zhang, Z. K. and Imperato-McGinley, J. L. 2005. Receptor isoform and ligand-specific modulation of dihydrotestosterone-induced prostate specific antigen gene expression and prostate tumor cell growth by estrogens. *J Androl*, 26(4): 500–508. discussion 509–510.

Chapter 5

ANTIOXIDANT PROPERTIES OF POMEGRANATES

ABSTRACT

Punica granatum L. (Punicaceae) is a deciduous shrub or small tree originally distributed in Iran and Afghanistan, and was introduced into China in the 2nd century BC. Pomegranate extracts have been shown to present potent antioxidant activity both *in vitro* and *in vivo* as well as numerous pharmacological activities that are vital for the therapeutic benefits of pomegranate consumption.

INTRODUCTION

Pomegranate juice is nutritionally an important beverage that is consumed frequently due to its rich polyphenolic content (such as anthocyanins, ellagic acid, phytoestrogenic flavonoids and tannins) [1]. Several studies have shown that pomegranate juice contains high levels of antioxidants – several fold greater than most other fruit juices and beverages. Recent clinical studies have shown that pomegranate juice reduces important blood parameters such as LDL, HDL, and cholesterol increase the prostate specific antigen (PSA), and may be protective against cardiovascular disease, cancers, neurodegenerative diseases, and infections [2]. Phenolic compounds such as major flavonoids and flavonoids are distributed throughout the pomegranate plant and contribute greatly to both the flavour and colour of pomegranates.

At present, there is a growing interest in identifying potent, naturally occurring antioxidants to minimize acute and chronic oxidative cellular damage. Oxidative damage caused by free radicals and reactive oxygen species occurs largely endogenously during key metabolic processes such as oxidative phosphorylation and ATP production. Different parts of the pomegranate fruit may exhibit important functional and medicinal effects such as antioxidant, anti-atherosclerotic, anti-cancer, neuroprotective and antimicrobial effects [3].

Flavonoids are C15 compounds containing 2 phenolic rings attached by a 3-carbon unit, and categorised based on their different substituents on the rings, and the degree of ring saturation. The presence of sugars moiety greatly increases their water-solubility. Flavonoids isolated from several parts of the pomegranate plant exhibit strong anti-oxidant activity. Phenolic compounds are a major determinant of antioxidant potentials of foods. Phenolic acid present in pomegranates consist of two subgroups; the hydroxybenzoic and hydroxycinnamic acids. Hydroxybenzoic acids include gallic, p-hydroxybenzoic, protocatechuic, vanillic and syringic acids, which in common have the C6–C1 structure. On the other hand, hydroxycinnamic acids, are aromatic compounds with a three-carbon side chain (C6–C3), with caffeic, ferulic, p-coumaric and sinapic acids being the most common [4].

Antioxidant Content of Pomegranates

Antioxidants from pomegranate leaf tissue have been isolated and identified and include flavone glycosides and gallo-and ellagitannins. The nutritional and antioxidant characteristics of pomegranate leaves have increased recent interest in their use as a beneficial source of secondary metabolites. As such, pomegranate leaves have been developed into a series of commercial products including green tea and other teas which are consumed in China, and have been included in nutrition capsules in the USA. Physical and chemical changes in pomegranate leaves have been reported [5].

The seasonal trends in nitrogen and carbohydrate contents in the leaves of 'Banati' pomegranate trees were studied during two successive growing seasons. The nitrogen content (% and mg/leaf) decreased gradually during the growing seasons of 1972 and 1973, while the total sugars (%) in the leaves fluctuated and did not show a discernable trend over the 2-year observation period. The starch content in the leaves tended to decrease from May to

August and then increased until the end of the growing season in both years (Lihua et al., 2010).

Pomegranate is a good example for this type of fruit. Pomegranate peels constitute approximately 40% of the whole fruit and are rich in ellagic acid derivatives such as the ellagitannins, punicalagin and penicillin. In addition, some ellagic acid derivatives (ellagic acid hexoside, -pentoside, etc.) are also present, although in lesser amounts. The most abundant of these polyphenols is punicalagin which is extracted from pomegranate juice during juice processing and which is responsible for more than 50% of the pomegranate juice's potent anti-oxidant activity [1-5].

The peel extracts of this plant had not significantly difference in ferrous reducing antioxidant power (FRAP) relative to aqueous juice difference was detected. The results showed that pomegranate juice of the malas variety had markedly higher antioxidant capacity than the other. The FRAP value of juice of three cultivars of pomegranate have been previously determined in an attempt to make a systematic comparison among their antioxidant activities. One study showed the content of flavonoids was higher in peel extract of wild soar variety than in malas pomegranate extract. The large amount of phenolic contained in peel extract may cause its strong antioxidant ability. Further studies on the effective antioxidants contained in these pomegranate juice and the mechanisms by which they protect against disease development are highly recommended [5].

Antioxidant Effects

Aviram et al., investigated the effect of 50 mL of pomegranate juice (equal to 1.5 mmol total polyphenols) in 13 healthy men age 20–35 years daily for 2 weeks. No significant differences in total, LDL, high-density-lipoprotein (HDL), or very-low-density-lipoprotein cholesterol levels or triglycerides were reported at the end of the study period. However, lipid peroxides decreased significantly by 6%. Antioxidant activity and serum paraoxonase concentration increased significantly by 9% ($p < 0.05$) and 18% ($p < 0.01$), respectively. Three patients were studied for an extended time period of ≤10 weeks and given increasing amounts of pomegranate juice, 20–80 mL daily (equal to 0.54–2.16 mmol total polyphenols). After week 1, lipid peroxide levels decreased by 11% with 20 mL of pomegranate juice daily. The amount of pomegranate juice was increased to 50 mL, which resulted in a 21%

decrease in lipid peroxide levels. Pomegranate juice amounts of over 50 mL daily did not result in further changes in lipid peroxide values. Platelet activation was decreased in platelet-rich plasma prepared from 11 volunteers who were given pomegranate juice for 2 weeks, demonstrated by an 11% decrease in collagen-induced platelet aggregation. However, the significance of the outcomes of this study is limited due to its small sample size, short duration, and lack of a control group [4].

Another study by Rosenblat et al. investigated the effects of pomegranate juice on oxidative stress and blood glucose levels in 10 adult men aged 35–71 years with type 2 diabetes mellitus. The study subjects were given 50 mL of pomegranate juice (equal to 1.5 mmol total polyphenols) daily for three months. The parameters for antioxidant activity were serum levels of lipid peroxides, paraoxonase 1, thiobarbituric acid reactive substances (TBARS), and total sulfhydryl groups. Paraoxonase 1 and total sulfhydryl groups exhibit antiatherosclerotic activity; lipid peroxides and TBARS exhibit oxidative activity. Total sulfhydryl groups are also a marker for oxidative stress. Levels of lipid peroxides and TBARS decreased by 56% and 28%, respectively ($p < 0.01$ for both) in this study. Total sulfhydryl groups and paraoxonase 1 levels increased by 12% and 24%, respectively ($p < 0.01$ for both). C-peptide levels (a product of proinsulin) decreased by 23%. Total cholesterol, LDL cholesterol, glycosylated hemoglobin, and triglycerides were not affected by pomegranate consumption. Insulin and glucose levels improved, but the differences were not significant. The authors concluded that pomegranate juice consumption did not worsen diabetes mellitus and exhibited antioxidant effects, which may attenuate atherosclerosis development; however, the applicability of these results is limited, because the study involved a small number of patients, was conducted for only three months, and involved surrogate markers [5].

The safety and efficacy of a pomegranate supplement was evaluated by Haber et al., in two studies. Patients were given a standardized, commercially available preparation, POMx (POM Wonderful, Los Angeles, CA), which is a pomegranate extract prepared from partially juice-pressed whole fruit and seeds (containing at least 90% polyphenols). All patients were overweight (body mass index of 25–32 kg/m^2), with a waist circumference of ≥35 inches for women or ≥40 inches for men, and treated for four weeks. In study 1, 64 patients age 35–65 years were given 710 mg of POMx, 1420 mg of POMx, or placebo daily in a capsule. Complete blood counts, blood chemistry values, urinalysis results, and vital signs were checked at three separate visits. There were no significant changes in laboratory values. No major adverse effects or allergic reactions were reported; however, 9 patients experienced minor adverse effects that the authors believed were unrelated to the pomegranate supplement. In study 2, 22 patients age 40–70 years were given two POMx capsules providing a total daily dose of 1000 mg of pomegranate. The mean ± S.D. TBARS concentration decreased by 0.13 ± 0.23 μM after POMx supplementation ($p = 0.044$). All other laboratory values remained unchanged; however, there was a significant increase in mean ± S.D. weight (1.30 ± 1.95 pounds, $p = 0.005$) that the authors believed was more likely a result of holiday-related eating than of the use of the pomegranate supplement. These studies were limited due to their short duration (four weeks). As well, the results may be specific to the POMx supplement used alone [6].

The antioxidant potential of pomegranate juice in comparison to apple juice was investigated by Guo et al. In this randomised study, 26 healthy Chinese patients over age 60 years were divided into two groups to receive apple or pomegranate juice. Apples are low in antioxidants, while pomegranates are high in antioxidants. Each patient consumed 250 mL of the assigned juice (the apple juice was a commercially available brand, whereas the pomegranate juice was a freshly squeezed preparation) daily for four weeks. Ferric-reducing antioxidant power (FRAP, which demonstrates antioxidant capacity), glutathione, ascorbic acid, and vitamin E levels were measured. The pomegranate juice group had a greater increase in the mean ± S.D. FRAP (1.46 ± 0.26 mmol/L) compared with the apple juice group (1.36 ± 0.14 mmol/L). There was no difference in glutathione, ascorbic acid, or vitamin E levels between groups. Consistent with the previous study, the results of this study need to be interpreted with caution due to its short duration and small sample size [7].

ANTIATHEROGENIC EFFECTS

The effects of pomegranate juice on ACE activity and blood pressure was evaluated by Aviram and Dornfeld in 10 hypertensive patients. Serum ACE activity and systolic blood pressure (SBP) were assessed before and after the patients ingested 50 mL of pomegranate juice (equal to 1.5 mmol total polyphenols) daily for two weeks. A 36% reduction in ACE activity and a 5% reduction in SBP (155 mm Hg before versus 147 mm Hg after, $p < 0.05$) were noted. The authors concluded that the significant reductions in ACE activity and SBP suggest that pomegranate juice may offer protection against some cardiovascular diseases; however, the results are limited because the study was not controlled, involved a small number of patients, and was only two weeks in duration [3].

The effects of pomegranate juice on carotid intima-media thickness (CIMT), blood pressure, and LDL oxidation was further investigated in atherosclerotic patients by Aviram et al. A total of 19 nonsmoking patients age 65–75 years who had asymptomatic severe carotid artery stenosis (70–90% stenosed) were randomized to receive either 50 mL of pomegranate juice (equal to 1.5 mmol total polyphenols) or placebo daily. All patients were followed for at least 1 year, and 5 of 10 patients in the pomegranate group were followed for 3 years. At 1 year, a mean decrease in CIMT of 35% occurred in the pomegranate group and an increase of 9% ($p < 0.01$) occurred in the placebo group. Further, SBP was significantly reduced by 12% in the pomegranate group (174 mm Hg pretreatment versus 153 mm Hg posttreatment, $p < 0.01$); no significant changes occurred in the placebo group (160 mm Hg pretreatment versus 163 mm Hg posttreatment). The concentration of antibodies against oxidized LDL was significantly reduced by 19% in the pomegranate group at three months ($p < 0.01$), and total serum antioxidants were increased by 130% in the pomegranate group at 1 year; no data were reported for the placebo group. No additional benefit was found in CIMT or SBP after 3 years; however, lipid peroxidation was further reduced. Although this study was limited by its small sample size and use of a surrogate marker, the authors concluded that pomegranate juice decreases progression of carotid lesions and SBP, possibly due to changes in oxidative stress [8].

Esmaillzadeh et al. investigated the effects of concentrated pomegranate juice on cholesterol levels in hyperlipidemic patients with type 2 diabetes mellitus. Twenty-two patients in Iran consumed 40 g of concentrated pomegranate juice (Nariran, Inc., Tehran, Iran) daily for two months. After treatment, patients' mean total cholesterol concentration decreased from 202 to 191 mg/dL ($p < 0.001$), mean LDL cholesterol concentration decreased from 123 to 112 mg/dL ($p < 0.006$), mean HDL cholesterol concentration remained unchanged (38 mg/dL), and mean triglyceride concentration decreased from 202 to 198 mg/dL (not statistically significant). The authors concluded that concentrated pomegranate juice may modify heart disease risk factors and be beneficial to include in balanced diets; however, the applicability of these results is limited, because the study did not have a control group, involved a small number of patients, and had a short duration [9].

Sumner et al. published a randomized, placebo-controlled, double-blind trial of the effects of pomegranate juice on myocardial perfusion in patients with coronary heart disease (CHD). Forty- five patients in the United States were randomized to receive either 240 mL of pomegranate juice (POM Wonderful) or a modified sports beverage of similar caloric content, flavor, and color daily for three months. The groups underwent exercise or pharmacologic (adenosine or dipyridamole) stress testing at baseline and three months. Stress-induced myocardial ischemia was quantified as the summed difference scores (SDS) and calculated by subtracting the summed rest score from the summed stress score. At three months, the mean ± S.D. SDS decreased in the pomegranate group by 0.8 ± 2.7 ($p < 0.05$) and increased in the control group by 1.2 ± 3.1 ($p < 0.05$); the difference between the groups was significant. Although the applicability of the study's results is limited by the small sample size and short duration, the authors concluded that daily consumption of pomegranate juice may improve stress-induced myocardial ischemia in patients with CHD [10].

Abidov et al. published a randomized, placebo-controlled, double-blind trial of the effects of Radical Fruits (Garden of Life, West Palm Beach, FL) on lipid concentrations. Forty-four non obese, nonsmoking, nondiabetic men with hypercholesterolemia were randomized to receive either 900 mg of Radical Fruits (a combination fruit supplement containing pomegranate juice) or placebo three times daily before meals for one month. Patients' baseline means total cholesterol, LDL cholesterol, and HDL cholesterol concentrations were measured. At the end of the trial, the treatment group had a reduction in mean total cholesterol concentration (from 280 to 250 mg/dL, $p < 0.001$), a reduction in LDL cholesterol concentration (from 195 to 169 mg/dL, $p < 0.001$), and an increase in HDL cholesterol concentration (from 49 to 52 mg/dL, $p < 0.001$). The placebo group experienced nonsignificant reductions in mean total cholesterol concentration (from 280 to 275 mg/dL), mean LDL cholesterol concentration (from 195 to 190 mg/dL), and HDL cholesterol concentration (from 49 to 48 mg/dL). The authors concluded that Radical Fruits may be effective for hypercholesterolemia and should be investigated in patients with cardiovascular disease. It is important to note that in addition to involving a small number of patients and having a short duration, this trial involved a product that contains a proprietary blend of many fruit supplements, so the effects cannot be attributed solely to pomegranate [11].

Davidson et al. published the results of a randomized, placebo-controlled, double-blind trial of pomegranate juice on CIMT progression. A total of 289 patients in the United States at moderate risk for CHD were randomized to receive either 240 mL of pomegranate juice (POM Wonderful) or a placebo beverage of similar caloric content and color daily for 18 months. The composite measurement of CIMT progression was smaller at 12 months in the pomegranate juice group compared with the placebo group (0.79 mm versus 0.81 mm, $p = 0.022$); however, the difference was not significant at 18 months (0.79 mm versus 0.80 mm, $p = 0.168$). In an exploratory analysis of the patients with the most adverse cardiovascular risk profiles, those in the pomegranate juice group had significantly less anterior wall or composite CIMT progression or both than did those in the placebo group. Although the study was limited by the use of a surrogate marker, the authors concluded that pomegranate juice consumption did not significantly reduce CIMT progression in patients at moderate risk for CHD but that it may slow progression in the subgroup of those patients at greatest risk [12].

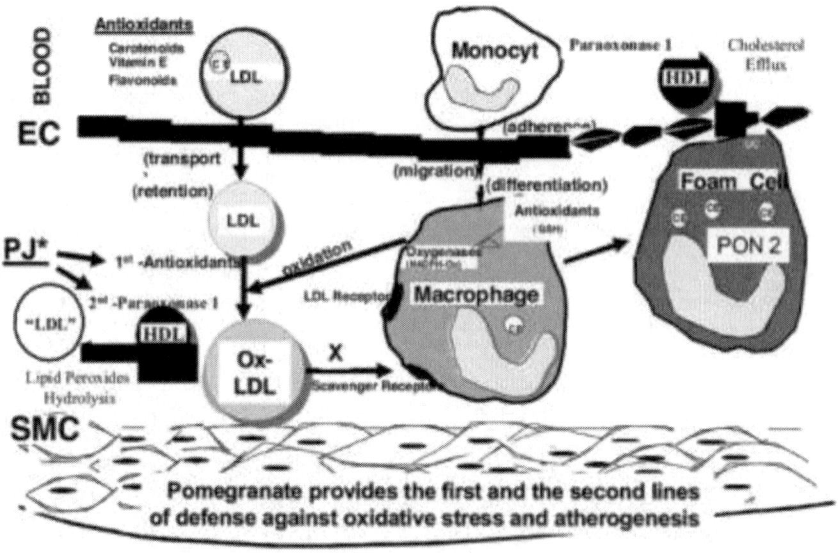

Figure 1. Antiatherogenic effect of pomegranates.

Future Prospects and Conclusion

The dosage of pomegranate used in the studies varied. Most provided 50 mL of juice daily (equal to 1.5 mmol total polyphenols); however, the quantities ranged from 20 to 250 mL. Also, some of the studies used a standardized, commercially available pomegranate preparation, while others used freshly squeezed juice [13-20]. The study that used POMx provided daily pomegranate doses of 710, 1000, and 1420 mg. The study that used Radical Fruits provided a daily dose of 900 mg. In another study, 40 g of pomegranate juice was given daily. In general, 50 mL of pomegranate juice daily is recommended for patients with hypertension and atherosclerosis. Dosages for patients with hyperlipidemia evaluated in the studies ranged from 900 mg to 40 g daily. The high levels of tannin in pomegranate may cause gastric irritation, and one study found a significant weight gain in patients who received a pomegranate supplement. Six publications described a total of 11 patients who developed allergic reactions, including pruritus, urticaria, angioedema, rhinorrhea, bronchospasm, dyspnea, and red itchy eyes, after ingesting pomegranate fruit [13–22]. One case report described contact urticaria syndrome of the allergic type in a woman who had been working with pomegranate seeds during the preparation of a meal. Patients with known allergic reactions to pomegranate, any of its constituents, or any of the plants in the punicaceae family should not ingest pomegranate. Dried pomegranate peel may contain aflatoxin, a potent hepatocarcinogen; thus, it should be used cautiously by patients who have hepatic dysfunction or who are taking other hepatotoxic agents.

References

[1] Natural Standard. Pomegranate (*Punica granatum*). www.naturalstandard.com (accessed 2010 Jun 28).

[2] Gruenwald J, Brendler T, Jaenicke C, eds. *PDR for herbal medicines. 4th ed.* Montvale, NJ: Thomson Healthcare Inc.; 2007.

[3] Aviram M, Dornfeld L. Pomegranate juice consumption inhibits serum angiotensin converting enzyme activity and reduces systolic blood pressure. *Atherosclerosis*. 2001; 158:195-8.

[4] Aviram M, Dornfeld L, Rosenblat M et al. Pomegranate juice consumption reduces oxidative stress, atherogenic modifications to LDL, and platelet aggregation: studies in humans and in atherosclerotic apolipoprotein E-deficient mice. *Am J Clin Nutr*. 2000; 71:1062-76.

[5] Rosenblat M, Hayek T, Aviram M. Antioxidant effects of pomegranate juice (PJ) consumption by diabetic patients on serum and on macrophages. *Atherosclerosis*. 2006; 187:363-71.

[6] Heber D, Seeram NP, Wyatt H et al. Safety and antioxidant activity of a pomegranate ellagitannin-enriched polyphenol dietary supplement in overweight individuals with increased waist size. *J Agric Food Chem.* 2007; 55:10050-4.

[7] Guo C, Wei J, Yang J et al. Pomegranate juice is potentially better than apple juice in improving antioxidant function in elderly subjects. *Nutr Res.* 2008; 28:72-7.

[8] Aviram M, Rosenblat M, Gaitini D et al. Pomegranate juice consumption for 3 years by patients with carotid artery stenosis reduces common carotid intimamedia thickness, blood pressure and LDL oxidation. *Clin Nutr.* 2004; 23:423-33.

[9] Esmaillzadeh A, Tahbaz F, Gaieni I et al. Concentrated pomegranate juice improves lipid profiles in diabetic patients with hyperlipidemia. *J Med Food.* 2004; 7:305-8.

[10] Sumner MD, Elliott-Eller M, Weidner G et al. Effects of pomegranate juice consumption in patients with coronary heart disease. *Am J Cardiol.* 2005; 96:810-4.

[11] Abidov M, Jimenez Del Rio M, Ramazanov A et al. Efficiency of pharmacologically active antioxidant phytomedicine Radical Fruits in treatment of hypercholesterolemia at men. *Georgian Med News.* 2006; 11:78-83.

[12] Davidson MH, Maki KC, Dicklin MR et al. Effects of consumption of pomegranate juice on carotid intima-media thickness in men and women at moderate risk for coronary heart disease. *Am J Cardiol.* 2009; 104:936-42.

[13] Igea JM, Cuesta J, Cuevas M et al. Adverse reaction to pomegranate ingestion. *Allergy.* 1991; 46:472-4.

[14] Gaig P, Botey J, Gutierrez V et al. Allergy to pomegranate (*Punica granatum*). *J Investig Allergol Clin Immunol.* 1992; 2:216-8.

[15] Gaig P, Bartolome B, Lleonart R et al. Allergy to pomegranate (*Punica granatum*). *Allergy.* 1999; 54:287-8.

[16] Enrique E, Utz M, De Mateo JA et al. Allergy to lipid transfer proteins: crossreactivity among pomegranate, hazelnut, and peanut. *Ann Allergy Asthma Immunol.* 2006; 96:122-3.

[17] Gangemi S, Mistrello G, Roncarlo D et al. Pomegranate-dependent exerciseinduced anaphylaxis. *J Investig Allergol Clin Immunol.* 2008; 18:491-2.

[18] Damiani E, Aloia AM, Priore MG et al. Pomegranate (*Punica granatum*) allergy: clinical and immunological findings. *Ann Allergy Asthma Immunol.* 2009; 103:178- 80.

[19] Valseechi R, Reseghetti A, Leghissa P et al. Immediate contact hypersensitivity to pomegranate. *Contact Dermatitis.* 1998; 38:44-5.

[20] Komperda KE. Potential interaction between pomegranate juice and warfarin. *Pharmacotherapy.* 2009; 29:1002-6.

[21] Farkas D, Oleson LE, Zhao Y et al. Pomegranate juice does not impair clearance of oral or intravenous midazolam, a probe for cytochrome P450-3A activity: comparison with grapefruit juice. *J Clin Pharmacol.* 2007; 47:286-94.

[22] Sorokin AV, Duncan B, Panetta R et al. Rhabdomyolysis associated with pomegranate juice consumption. *Am J Cardiol.* 2006; 98:705-6.

Chapter 6

Protection against Cardiovascular Diseases

Abstract

Cardiovascular disease ranks among the leading causes of morbidity and mortality in adults in the developed world. While improved diet and lifestyle modification such as regular physical activity are the primary preventive health approaches, there is an increasing role for the use of bioactive phytochemicals as therapeutic agents due to their unique protective benefits on the cardiovascular system. Pomegranates are polyphenol-rich fruits which possess potent antioxidant capacity. Several *in vitro* and *in vivo* studies have demonstrated significant antiatherogenic, antioxidant, antihypertensive and anti-inflammatory effects of pomegranate consumption. Pomegranates have been shown to reduce the size of atherosclerotic plaques in mice models, and reduced lipid peroxidation in human patients with type 2 non-insulin dependent diabetes, and systolic blood pressure, in hypertensive patients. Thus the protective effects of pomegranates on cardiovascular disease warrants further investigation, and growing evidence suggests that it wise to incorporate pomegranates in a cardioprotective diet.

Introduction

Several epidemiological studies have shown that a diet rich in fruits and vegetables are associated with a significantly lowered risk of coronary heart disease (CHD) and stroke. Fruits and vegetables are composed of a wide array of important phytochemicals, including carotenoids, and major polyphenolic compounds such as flavonoids, resveratrol, tannins, isothiocyanates and organosulfur compounds, which have been shown to attenuate or at least slow down the pathogenesis of several cardiovascular diseases both *in vivo* and *in vitro*. The beneficial effects of fruits and vegetables stems from the combination of phytochemicals, fibres and other vitamins and nutrients, rather than the biological activity of individual components alone. It is well established that phytochemicals display potent antioxidant and anti-inflammatory properties which counteract oxidative damage and inflammation which play a major role in the aetiology and development of cardiovascular diseases. There is a growing emphasis to not only consume nine servings of fruits and vegetables daily, but also to understand the vital benefits of consuming specific phytochemical-rich fruits and vegetable with protective effects on cardiovascular disease [1-5].

Atherosclerosis, Oxidative Stress and Inflammation

Atherosclerosis represents the most common type of coronary artery disease. Morphologically, atherosclerosis is characterised by the accumulation of fatty streak composed of lipid-filled (mainly cholesterol and cholesterol esters) foam cells, the presumed precursor lesion for atheromas. An atheroma or atheromatous plaque consists of a raised focal lesion that proceeds in the intima of the vessel wall leading to the formation of fatty/fibrous plaques and abnormal calcium deposition. The interior of the affected vessel may be blocked by fatty plaques, which causes thickening and loss of elasticity in the vessel wall. The atheromatous plaque may appear as white to whitish yellow, and impinge on the lumen of the artery. It may vary in size, ranging from 0.3 to 1.5 cm in diameter, but may coalesce to form larger masses. Atherosclerotic lesions are located partially around the circumference of the arterial wall, and distributed variably along the vessel length. Initially focal and sparsely distributed, atherosclerotic lesions become more and more numerous and diffuse as the disease progresses. Over time, plaques may lose their surface; leading to blood coagulates to form on them. This effect is known a thrombus formation, and may further contribute to obstruction the coronary arteries (known as coronary heart disease). Several lines of evidence suggest that obesity, hypertension, diabetes mellitus, dyslipidaemia, smoking, advanced ageing, diets rich in saturated fats and reduced physical activity increase the risk of atherosclerosis, which is also characterised by extensive oxidative stress and inflammation [6-10].

Atherosclerotic plaques are more dominantly distributed in the abdominal aorta than the thoracic aorta, with lesions more commonly localised around the origins (Ostia) of major branches. After the lower abdominal aorta, the most extensively inflicted vessels are the coronary arteries and the popliteal arteries, the internal carotid arteries and the vessels of the circle of Willis. Vessels in the upper extremities are least affected, as are the mesenteric and renal arteries, except at their Ostia. However, the severity of atherosclerosis present in one artery plays no causal effect on atherosclerotic severity in another artery [11-15].

Atherosclerotic plaques are composed of three key components: (1) several cell varieties, including smooth muscle cells (SMCs), macrophages, and other leukocytes; (2) extracellular matrix containing collagen, elastic fibres, and proteoglycans; and (3) intracellular and extracellular lipids. While the proportion of these components varies in different lesions, the superficial fibrous cap is typically composed of SMCs and thick collagen. Underneath the cap (otherwise known as the 'shoulder') is a cellular area populated with macrophages, SMCs, and T lymphocytes. Deeper within the plaque is a necrotic core containing deregulated lipids such as cholesterol and cholesterol esters, debris from apoptotic cells, foam cells, fibrin, variably organised thrombus and other plasma protein [16-19].

Oxidative stress plays a significant contribution to the development of cardiovascular disease, an inflammation as a manifestation of oxidative stress. Oxidative stress occurs in response to an imbalance in the formation of free radicals, and the body's endogenous antioxidant status. Oxidative stress can promote inflammation by activating a variety of cellular pathways that produce inflammatory mediators such as cell adhesion molecules, and pro-inflammatory cytokines. Numerous human studies have identified a strong correlation between increased oxidative stress and inflammation, and increased vascular damage such as endothelial dysfunction, elevated arterial stiffness, platelet activation, and angiogenesis. Vascular SMC activation and proliferation is mediated by oxidative stress and inflammation. Several biomarkers of inflammation are elevated in cardiovascular diseases. These include C-reactive protein (CRP), vascular cell adhesion molecule-1 (VCAM-1), tumour necrosis factor-α (TNF-α), interleukin-1 (IL-1), interleukin-18 (IL-18), soluble CD40 ligand (sCD40L), and monocyte matrix metalloproteinase 9 (MMP-9). Oxidative biomarkers for cardiovascular diseases include increased levels of lipid peroxidation markers such as 4-hydroxynonenal (4-HNE), oxidised-low-density-lipoprotein (LDL), and urinary 8-isoprostane levels [20-25].

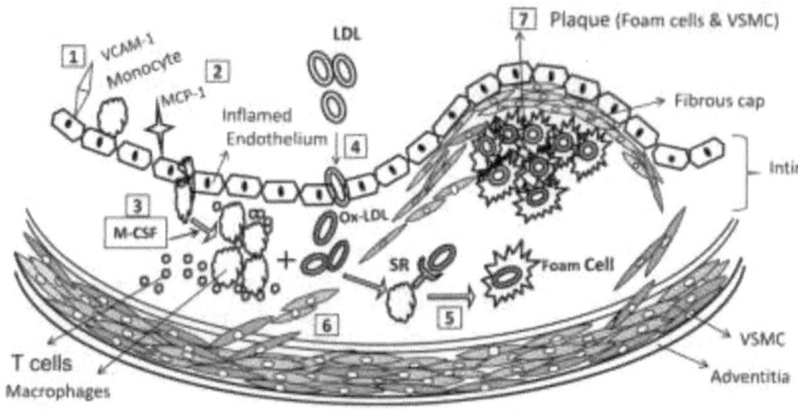

Figure 1. Pathobiology of Atherosclerosis.

Impaired endothelial function occurs in response to reduced nitric oxide (NO) bioavailability due to increased formation of peroxynitrate, which can induce cell death via energy restriction and apoptosis. During inflammation, endothelial cells express VCAM-1 and promote adhesion of monocytes, and early step in the pathogenesis of atherosclerosis. Increased expression of selectins, integrins, and monocyte chemoattractant protein-1 (MCP-1) in endothelial cells, stimulate the migration of monocytes into the vulnerable intima, where they will remain and multiply. The consequent inflammation in the intima triggers the production of macrophage colony stimulating factor (M-CSF) which induces monocytes to mature into macrophages. Afterwards, atherogenic lipoproteins such as LDL and very low density lipoprotein (VLDL) accumulate in the subintimal space where they can undergo oxidative modifications leading to the formation of oxidised LDL. Mature macrophages develop scavenger receptors capable of phagocytising oxidised LDL to form lipid-filled foam cells whilst also secreting major proinflammatory cytokines such as TNF-α, and IL-1β. This process is followed by increased VSMC migration and proliferation mediated by both T-cells and residing migration and proliferation. The last stage is mediated by the expression of specific enzymes in VSMC that break down collagen, and weaken the fibrous cap of the atheroma, making it susceptible to rupture. Marked inflammation stimulates the release of pro-coagulent factors, which induces the thrombosis and plaque ruptures. As oxidative stress and inflammation are pivotal events in pathogenesis of atherosclerosis and other related cardiovascular disorders, strategies aimed at preserving the endothelium by attenuating oxidative stress and inflammation are warranted [26-30].

CLINICAL APPLICATIONS OF POMEGRANATES IN CARDIOVASCULAR DISEASE

Atherosclerosis

Several *in vitro* and *in vivo* studies using extensive animal models and human clinical trials have examined the effects of several pomegranate constituents on prevention and protection against atherosclerosis. One study investigated the effects of pomegranate juice and other polyphenolic rich fruit juices on endothelial function. In particular, the study focussed on comparing propensities to protect endothelial cells against NO and free-radical mediated destruction. Results of the antioxidant portion of the study showed that pomegranate juice contains a significantly greater antioxidant capacity at relatively lower concentrations (>1000-fold dilutions) compared to either grape or blueberry juice. This is related to the higher amounts of anthocyanin flavonoid content and total flavonoid content in pomegranate juice than the other juices.

As mentioned earlier, impaired endothelial function is an early indicator of atherosclerosis. One important study examined the effect of pomegranate juice on the proliferation of rat aortic smooth muscle cells in culture. This study showed that pomegranate juice significantly enhances the effect of NO on the cardiac endothelium at up to 2,000-fold dilutions compared to other juices. Interestingly, pomegranate juice was unable to affect the expression of endothelial nitric oxide synthase (eNOS). The authors suggested that the antioxidant properties of pomegranate juice are likely to protect NO from oxidative insult and augment the antiproliferative action of NO on rat aortic smooth muscle cells [35-38].

The early-stage atherosclerosis has been reported to involve elevated plasma Cholesterol, increased oxidative stress and increased cholesterol esterification that contributes to the formation of foam cells, and the development and progression of the atherosclerotic plaque. Moreover, pomegranate extracts have been shown to inhibit atherogenesis in atherosclerotic apolipoprotein-E deficient (E°) mice. Consumption of pomegranate juice to E° mice with advanced atherosclerosis for two months showed a 42% reduction in lipid peroxide content in mouse peritoneal macrophages (MPM) compared to placebo-treated mice. Similarly, the MPM lipid peroxide content in PJ-treated mice was 20% lower than in four-month-old wild-type control mice. The same study further demonstrated that MPM harvested from PJ-treated mice contained 80% lower rates of cholesterol esterification compared to placebo-treated mice. As well, the size of atherosclerotic lesions in the aorta was reduced by 17% compared to the age-matched placebo group [39-40].

Additionally, pomegranate juice and an isolated tannin fraction extracted from pomegranate juice were also given to young E° mice prior to the development of significant atherosclerosis. The results showed about 25% reductions in plasma lipid peroxide concentrations with the isolated tannins, and 17% with the pomegranate juice. This suggests that the cardioprotective effect of pomegranates may be due to specific tannins present in the fruit [41-43].

Another study of four-month-old E° mice with significant atherosclerosis, pomegranate extract containing 51.5μg gallic acid equiv/kg/day). The study reported an eight-fold higher polyphenol concentration than pomegranate juice alone for three months. The results also showed a significant reduction in MPM oxidative status as measured by a 27% decrease in total macrophage peroxide levels, a 42% decrease in cellular lipid peroxide levels, and a 19% decrease in peritoneal macrophage uptake of oxidized LDL [31-34].

The key question is which part of the fruit contains the most potent antiatherogenic compounds. To answer this question, one study fed atherosclerotic E° mice with six different pomegranate preparations with varying amounts of total polyphenols and gallic acid content for three months. Antioxidant activity, atherosclerotic lesion size, MPM oxidative status, blood sugar and lipid profiles were examined. Consistent with earlier results, the study demonstrated that pomegranate flower extract most significantly reduced atherosclerotic lesion size, lipid profiles, and blood sugar levels than other extracts tested. On the contrary, two pomegranate pulp extracts demonstrated the most potent antioxidant effects. Mechanisms associated with the anti-atherogenic effects of pomegranate in this study include increased MPM uptake of oxidized LDL, decreased lipid peroxidation and decreased cholesterol levels [44-47].

The effect of pomegranate juice consumption on lipid peroxidation and the levels of plasma and HDL- and LDL-lipoproteins have also been previously investigated in a double-armed human trial. In the first study, 13 healthy, non-smoking men (ages 20-35) were given 50 mL pomegranate juice daily (containing 1.5 mmol total polyphenols) for two weeks. In the second study (duration ≤10 weeks), three healthy men (same age range) were given increasing doses of pomegranate juice ranging from 20-80 mL daily (0.54-2.16 mmol total polyphenols). Fasting blood samples were collected from participants pre-study, and after one and two weeks of PJ supplementation. On the contrary to previous animal studies, the human trial found no significant effect on plasma lipid profile or lipoprotein patterns. However, the results are the first to show that pomegranate juice has an inhibitory effect on lipid peroxidation in plasma and in lipoproteins in humans. An effective dose of 50 mL daily yielded a 32% decrease in plasma lipid peroxidation. Supplementation with pomegranate juice also demonstrated up to 90% reduction in collagen-induced platelet aggregation in human platelets *ex vivo* in a dose dependent manner [48-50].

Hyperlipidemia

Hyperlipidemia is a major risk factor for ischemic heart disease and impaired coronary function. There is a strong correlation between enhanced platelet activity, high LDL cholesterol levels and low platelet reactivity with low cholesterol levels. Therefore, strategies aimed at lowering blood cholesterol levels can reduce cardiovascular events.

Pomegranate flowers have been traditionally used in both the Unani and Ayurvedic systems of medicine as a natural treatment for diabetes mellitus. Considering the historical use of pomegranates, one study examined the effects of pomegranate flower extract on cardiac lipid metabolism in 13-to 15-week old Zucker diabetic rats. These rodents were fed 500 mg/kg of pomegranate flower extract or placebo for six weeks. The parameters that were assessed were total cholesterol, triglyceride, and nonesterified free fatty acids (NEFA) prior to treatment, after 4 weeks treatment, in both rat plasma and cardiac tissue. The pomegranate flower extract was shown to activate peroxisome proliferator-activated receptor (PPAR), a well-established cardiac transcription factor associated with myocardial energy production via fatty acid uptake and oxidation. Activation of PPAR reduced cardiac uptake and circulation of lipids. The total cardiac tissue triglyceride content, and plasma total cholesterol was also reduced at the end of the study [52-58].

Another pilot study comprised of 22 type 2 diabetic patients (8 men and 14 women) investigated the cholesterol-lowering effects of 40 g concentrated pomegranate juice for eight weeks. The study found statistically significant decreases were in total cholesterol (from 202.4 mg/dL at baseline to 191.4 mg/dL at study conclusion), LDL cholesterol (124.4 mg/dL at baseline to 112.9 mg/dL at study conclusion), total/HDL cholesterol ratio (5.5 at baseline to 5.1 at study conclusion), and LDL/HDL ratio (3.4 at baseline to 3.0 at study conclusion). The authors attributed these effects to decreased absorption and increased faecal excretion of cholesterol, as well as possible effects on HMG-CoA reductase and sterol O-acyltransferase, two enzymes key to cholesterol metabolism [59-60].

Hypertension

At least 970 million people worldwide suffer from elevated blood pressure or hypertension. Hypertension represents the major cause of premature death worldwide and the problem is increasing significantly. It is a major risk factor for coronary heart disease and the single most important risk factor for stroke. It has been estimated that over 1.56 billion adults will be diagnosed with hypertension in 2025.

Increased blood pressure is defined as a systolic blood pressure at above 140 mmHg and/or diastolic blood pressure at or above 90 mmHg. Systolic blood pressure is defined as the maximum pressure in arteries when the heart contracts. Diastolic blood pressure is defined as the minimum pressure in the arteries between the heart's contractions. Hypertension can stress the body's vasculature, leading to vessel weakness. Hypertension can lead to atherosclerosis and narrowing of blood vasculature making them more prone to blockage due to the formation of thrombi or fatty streaks. Extensive damage to arteries can also lead to the formation of irregular vascular projections known as aneurisms [61]

While increased blood pressure is thought to occur as part of the ageing process, several strategies have been identified aimed at reducing the risk. These include a healthy, relatively low salt diet, physical activity and reduced calorie intake. One pilot study showed that pomegranate juice can reduce systolic blood pressure in hypertensive patients. Ten hypertensive subjects (ages 62-77; seven men and three women) were given 50 mL/ day PJ containing 1.5 mmol total polyphenols for two weeks. Two of seven patients were also diabetic and two were hyperlipidaemia. Seven of 10 subjects (70%) experienced a significant, five % decrease in systolic blood pressure [62-67].

Carotid Artery Stenosis

The narrowing of the lumen of the carotid artery is known as carotid artery stenosis and usually occurs due to atherosclerosis. The carotid artery projects from the brachiocephalic trunk as the common carotid artery, and on the left side the common carotid artery comes directly off the aortic arch. At the throat it forks into the internal and external carotid arteries. The internal carotid artery supplies the brain, and the external carotid artery supplies the face. This fork is a common site for atherosclerosis, an inflammatory buildup of athermanous plaque that can narrow the lumen of the common or internal carotid arteries.

The plaque can be stable and asymptomatic, or it can be a source of embolization. Emboli break off from the plaque and travel through the circulation to blood vessels in the brain. As the vessel gets smaller they can lodge in the vessel wall and restrict blood flow to parts of the brain which that vessel supplies. This ischemia can either be temporary, yielding a transient ischemic attack, or permanent resulting in a thromboembolic stroke. Transient ischemic attacks (TIA's) are a warning sign, and are often followed by severe permanent strokes, particularly within the first two days. TIA's by definition last less than 24 hours and frequently take the form of a weakness or loss of sensation of a limb or the trunk on one side of the body, or the loss of sight (amaurosis fugax) in one eye. Less common symptoms are artery sounds (bruits), or ringing in the ears (tinnitus).

In a small, long-term study involving 19 subjects aged between 65-75, with severe carotid artery stenosis (70-90% stenosis of internal carotid arteries), subjects were randomized to receive either 50 mL pomegranate juice daily containing 1.5 mmoles total polyphenols (n=10) or no placebo (n=9) for one year. Five subjects continued treatment with pomegranate juice for an additional two years. Study participants were treated with similar hypocholesterolemic and antihypertensive medications and no dietary or lifestyle changes occurred in either group. Blood samples were collected and echo Doppler analysis was performed at baseline and at 3, 6, 9, 12, 22, 28, and 36 months. Control subjects demonstrated a mean 9% increase in intima-media thickness (IMT) of left and right carotid arteries during the first year. Conversely, that consuming pomegranate juice had reduced IMT at 3, 6, 9, and

12 months ranging from 13% at three months to 35 percent at one year compared to baseline values [63-69].

With the exception of serum triglyceride concentrations, major serum biomarkers remained unchanged following pomegranate juice consumption during the first year. Serum triglyceride levels increased up to 16% but remained within the normal range. Pomegranate juice consumption also significantly reduced serum lipid peroxidation by 59% after one year, and levels of LDL-associated lipid peroxides were also markedly reduced by 90% after 6 months of supplementation. Body mass index remained unchanged in treated subjects but systolic blood pressure was lowered by 16% during the entire 3 year duration of the study. Apart from previous studies showing the effect of reduced systolic blood pressure and inhibition of lipid peroxidation due to pomegranate juice, this study provided first-hand evidence to suggest that pomegranate consumption can significantly reduce several aspects of IMT in patients with severe carotid artery stenosis via antioxidant mechanisms [70-73].

Myocardial Infarction

Myocardial infarction, or acute myocardial infarction (AMI, is the medical term for an event commonly known as a heart attack. AMI occurs when blood stops flowing properly to part of the heart and the heart muscle is injured or becomes hypoxic due to not receiving enough oxygen. This occurs as a response to blockage of at least one of the coronary arteries that supply blood to the heart. Blockage is likely to arise due to an unstable buildup of white blood cells, cholesterol and/or fat.

Symptoms of acute MI usually involve sudden acute chest pain that is felt behind the breast bone and may extend to the left arm or the left side of the neck. Additional symptoms may include shortness of breath, sweating, nausea, vomiting, abnormal heartbeats, and anxiety. These symptoms are less likely to occur in women than men. Up to 64% of people do not experience chest pain or other symptoms, and this is known as "silent" myocardial infarctions.

Important risk factors include previous cardiovascular disease, old age, tobacco smoking, high blood levels of certain lipids (low-density lipoprotein cholesterol, triglycerides) and low levels of high density lipoprotein (HDL) cholesterol, diabetes, hypertension, lack of physical activity, obesity, chronic kidney disease, excessive alcohol consumption, and the use of cocaine and amphetamines. The most common triggering event is the disruption of an atherosclerotic plaque in an epicardia coronary artery, which activates a clotting cascade, culminating in total occlusion of the artery. When a severe enough plaque rupture occurs in the coronary vasculature, it leads to MI (necrosis of downstream myocardium).

If blood flow to the heart is impaired for a long period of time, it triggers a process known as ischemia. In this process, myocardial cells located in the precinct of the occluded coronary artery become necrotic and cannot regenerate. A collagen scar forms in their place. Recent studies have shown that apoptosis may also play a role in the process of tissue damage subsequent to MI. As a result, the patient's heart will be permanently damaged. This myocardial scarring also puts the patient at risk for potentially life-threatening arrhythmias, and may result in the formation of a ventricular aneurysm that can rupture with catastrophic consequences.

The conduction of electrical impulses is slower in the injured heart than in normal heart tissue. The difference in conduction velocity between injured and uninjured tissue can trigger re-entry or a feedback loop that is believed to be the cause of many lethal arrhythmias. Atherosclerosis is the primary cause of myocardial infarction. Inflammation and oxidative stress may a major role in the pathogenesis and development of MI. Elevated CRP blood levels, especially measured with high-sensitivity assays, are predictive of the risk of MI, as well as stroke and development of diabetes.

In a double-blind, randomized, placebo-controlled trial, 39 patients were given either 240 mL pomegranate juice (n=23) or a sports beverage of similar colour, flavour, and caloric content daily for three months (n=16). While both control and treatment patients demonstrated similar levels of stress-induced ischemia at baseline, stress-induced ischemia was increased after 3 months in the placebo group (from 5.9 to 7.1) but reduced in the treatment group (from 4.5 to 3.7). Similarly, the rate of angina episodes increased to 38% in the placebo group but decreased sharply by 50% in the treatment group. These results demonstrate a significant reduction in myocardial ischemia in patients consuming pomegranate juice [74-76].

Diabetes

Diabetes mellitus (DM) also simply known as diabetes, is a major metabolic disorder where blood sugar levels are significantly elevated over a prolonged period of time. Increased glucose levels lead to symptoms of frequent urination, increased thirst, and increased hunger. If left untreated, diabetes can cause many complications, including diabetic ketoacidosis and nonketotic hyperosmolar coma. Serious long-term complications include cardiovascular disease, stroke, kidney failure, foot ulcers and ocular damage.

Diabetes is due to either the pancreas not producing enough insulin, or the cells of the body not being able to respond appropriately to the insulin that is produced. There are three main types of diabetes mellitus: (1) Type 1 DM occurs when the body is unable to produce enough insulin. This form was previously referred to as "insulin-dependent diabetes mellitus" (IDDM) or "juvenile diabetes", and has an unknown etiology. (2) Type 2 DM occurs due to the development of insulin resistance, a condition in which cells fail to respond to insulin properly. As the disease progresses a lack of insulin may also develop. This form was previously referred to as non-insulin-dependent diabetes mellitus (NIDDM) or "adult-onset diabetes". Increased body weight and not enough exercise are the main risk factors for Type 2 DM. (3) Gestational diabetes is the third main form and occurs in pregnant women without a previous history of diabetes and who develop a high blood glucose level.

Prevention and treatment involves consuming healthy diet, physical exercise, abstaining from tobacco smoking and maintaining a normal body weight. Maintaining a normal blood pressure is also important for people with the disease. Type 1 diabetes is almost always managed with insulin injections. Type 2 diabetes may be treated with medications with or without insulin injections depending on the severity of the disorder. Gestational diabetes usually resolves after the birth of the baby.

Globally, as of 2013, an estimated 382 million people have been diagnosed with diabetes worldwide, with type 2 diabetes accounting for almost 90% of all cases. This is equal to 8.3% of the adult population, with equal rates in both women and men. Worldwide in 2012 and 2013 diabetes resulted in 1.5 to 5.1 million deaths per year, making it the 8th leading cause of death. Diabetes overall at least doubles the risk of death. The number of people with diabetes is expected to rise to 592 million by 2035. The economic costs of diabetes globally were estimated in 2013 at $548 billion and in the United States in 2012 $245 billion.

In an animal model of diabetes, Huang et al. showed that pomegranate flower extract can maintain plasma lipid profiles and attenuate cardiac fibrosis in Zucker fatty diabetic rats. Rosenblat et al. further demonstrated that 50 mL/day of pomegranate juice for three months could reduce oxidative stress, blood sugar levels, and maintain normal healthy lipid profiles in 10 type 2 diabetic patients (history of diabetes for 4-10 years) and 10 healthy controls (ages 35-71). In diabetic patients, triglyceride levels were 2.8 times greater, HDL cholesterol was 28-percent lower, and haemoglobin A1C (HbA1C) values were 59-percent higher than in control patients. Insulin was only slightly lower in patients than controls, and C-peptide (a proinsulin metabolite marker for endogenously secreted insulin) was slightly higher in diabetic patients than in healthy controls at baseline (indicating slight hyperinsulinemia). Pomegranate juice consumption for three months did not significantly affect triglyceride, HDL cholesterol, HbA1C, glucose, or insulin values, but did lower serum C-peptide values by 23 percent compared to baseline in diabetic patients – a sign of improved insulin sensitivity [77-80].

Pomegranate juice consumption also significantly reduced oxidative stress in the diabetic patients as evidenced by a 56% reduction in lipid peroxides compared to baseline serum levels. The study also showed a 39% decrease in uptake of oxidized LDL by human monocyte-derived macrophages (an early development in foam cell formation and atherogenesis during atherosclerosis) was observed in diabetic patients following consumption of pomegranate juice. The study suggested that despite the sugars naturally present in pomegranate juice, consumption of this drink did not adversely affect parameters for diabetes and atherosclerosis [80-84].

Future Prospects and Conclusion

Pomegranate and its constituents have safely been consumed for centuries without adverse effects. Studies of pomegranate constituents in animals at concentrations and levels commonly used in folk and traditional medicine note no toxic effects. Toxicity of the polyphenol antioxidant punicalagin, abundant in pomegranate juice, was evaluated in rats. No toxic effects or significant differences histopathological analysis of rat organs. Research in 86 overweight human volunteers demonstrated the safety of a tableted PFE in amounts up to 1,420 mg/day (870 mg gallic acid equivalents) for 28 days, with no adverse events reported or adverse changes in blood or urine laboratory values observed.93 Another study in 10 patients with carotid artery stenosis demonstrated PJ consumption (121 mg/L EA equivalents) for up to three years had no toxic effect on blood chemistry analysis for kidney, liver, and heart function were observed in the treatment group compared to controls, which was confirmed via An explosion of interest in the numerous therapeutic properties of *Punica granatum* over the last decade has led to numerous *in vitro*, animal, and clinical trials. Pomegranate is a potent antioxidant, superior to red wine and equal to or better than green tea. In addition, its potent anti-inflammatory properties suggest its possible use as a therapy or adjunct for prevention and treatment of several types of cardiovascular disease.

References

[1] Kung HC, Hoyert DL, Xu J, Murphy SL. Deaths: final data for 2005. *Natl Vital Stat Rep*. 2008;56:1–120.

[2] Burrows NR, Parekh S, Li Y, Geiss LS. Prevalence of selfreported cardiovascular disease among persons aged _35 years with diabetes – United States, 1997–2005. *MMWR*. 2007;56:1129–1131. Available at: http://www.cdc.gov/mmwr/preview/mmwrhtml/mm5643a2.htm. Accessed 25 July 2008.

[3] Ruel G, Couillard C. Evidences of the cardioprotective potential of fruits: the case of cranberries. *Mol Nutr Food Res*. 2007;51:692–701.

[4] Kuriyama S. The relation between green tea consumption and cardiovascular disease as evidenced by epidemiological studies. *J Nutr*. 2008;138(Suppl):S1548–S1553.

[5] Hooper L, Kroon PA, Rimm EB, et al. Flavonoids, flavonoid-rich foods, and cardiovascular risk: a meta-analysis of randomized controlled trials. *Am J Clin Nutr*. 2008;88:38–50.

[6] Kris-Etherton PM, Lefevre M, Beecher GR, Gross MD, Keen CL, Etherton TD. Bioactive compounds in nutrition and healthresearch methodologies for establishing biological function: the antioxidant and anti-inflammatory effects of flavonoids on atherosclerosis. *Annu Rev Nutr*. 2004;24:511–538.

[7] Law MR, Morris JK. By how much does fruit and vegetable consumption reduce the risk of ischaemic heart disease? *Eur J Clin Nutr*. 1998;52:549–556.

[8] Joshipura KJ, Hu FB, Manson JE, et al. The effect of fruit and vegetable intake on risk for coronary heart disease. *Ann Intern Med*. 2001;34:1106–1114.

[9] Joshipura KJ, Ascherio A, Manson JE, et al. Fruit and vegetable intake in relation to risk of ischemic stroke. *JAMA*. 1999;282:1233–1239.

[10] Iribarren C, Folsom AR, Jacobs DR Jr, Gross MD, Belcher JD, Eckfeldt JH. Association of serum vitamin levels, LDL susceptibility to oxidation, and autoantibodies against MDA-LDL with carotid atherosclerosis. A case-control study. The ARIC Study Investigators.

Atherosclerosis risk in communities. *Arterioscler Thromb Vasc Biol.* 1997;17:1171–1177.

[11] Sesso HD, Buring JE, Norkus EP, Gaziano JM. Plasma lycopene, other carotenoids, and retinol and the risk of cardiovascular disease in women. *Am J Clin Nutr.* 2004;79:47–53.

[12] Erlund I, Koli R, Alfthan G, et al. Favorable effects of berry consumption on platelet function, blood pressure, and HDL cholesterol. *Am J Clin Nutr.* 2008;87:323–331.

[13] Fukao H, Ijiri Y, Miura M, et al. Effect of trans-resveratrol on the thrombogenicity and atherogenicity in apolipoprotein E-deficient and low-density lipoprotein receptor-deficient mice. *Blood Coagul Fibrinolysis.* 2004;15:441–446.

[14] Heber D, Seeram NP, Wyatt H, et al. Safety and antioxidant activity of a pomegranate ellagitannin-enriched polyphenol dietary supplement in overweight individuals with increased waist size. *J Agric Food Chem.* 2007;55:10050–10054.

[15] Nettleton JA, Steffen LM, Mayer-Davis EJ, et al. Dietary patterns are associated with biochemical markers of inflammation and endothelial activation in the Multi-Ethnic Study of Atherosclerosis (MESA). *Am J Clin Nutr.* 2006;83:1369–1379.

[16] Ackermann RT, Mulrow CD, Ramirez G, et al. Garlic shows promise for improving some cardiovascular risk factors. *Arch Intern Med.* 2001;161:813–824.

[17] Tipoe GL, Leung TM, Hung MW, Fung ML. Green tea polyphenols as an anti-oxidant and anti-inflammatory agent for cardiovascular protection. *Cardiovasc Hematol Disord Drug Targets.* 2007;7:135–144.

[18] Cho SY, Park SJ, Kwon MJ, et al. Quercetin suppresses proinflammatory cytokine production through MAP kinases and NF-kappaB pathway in lipopolysaccharide-stimulated macrophage. *Mol Cell Biochem.* 2003;243:153–160.

[19] Bhatt DL. Anti-inflammatory agents and antioxidants as a possible "third great wave" in cardiovascular secondary prevention. *Am J Cardiol.* 2008;101:4D–13D.

[20] Basu A, Lucas EA. Mechanisms and effects of green tea on cardiovascular health. *Nutr Rev.* 2007;65:361–375.

[21] U.S. Department of Agriculture (USDA). U.S. Department of Health and Human Services. *Dietary Guidelines for Americans 2005. Food Groups to Encourage.* Available at: http:// www.health.gov/dietaryguidelines/ dga2005/document/html/chapter5.htm. Accessed 28 July 2008.

[22] Seeram NP. Berry fruits: compositional elements, biochemical activities, and the impact of their intake on human health, performance, and disease. *J Agric Food Chem*. 2008;56:627– 629.

[23] Aviram M, Rosenblat M, Gaitini D, et al. Pomegranate juice consumption for 3 years by patients with carotid artery stenosis reduces common carotid intima-media thickness, blood pressure and LDL oxidation. *Clin Nutr*. 2004;23:423– 433.

[24] Sumner MD, Elliott-Eller M, Weidner G, et al. Effects of pomegranate juice consumption on myocardial patients with coronary heart disease. *Am J Cardiol*. 2005;96:810–814.

[25] Chun OK, Chung SJ, Claycombe KJ, Song WO. Serum C-reactive protein concentrations are inversely associated with dietary flavonoid intake in U.S. adults. *J Nutr*. 2008;138:753–760.

[26] Ellingsen I, Hjerkinn EM, Seljeflot I, Arnesen H, Tonstad S. Consumption of fruit and berries is inversely associated with carotid therosclerosis in elderly men. *Br J Nutr*. 2008;99:674– 681.

[27] Fan J, Watanabe T. Inflammatory reactions in the pathogenesis of atherosclerosis. *J Atheroscler Thromb*. 2003;10:63–71.

[28] Holvoet P. Relations between metabolic syndrome, oxidative stress and inflammation and cardiovascular disease [in Dutch]. *Verh K Acad Geneeskd Belg*. 2008;70:193–219.

[29] Kals J, Kampus P, Kals M, et al. Inflammation and oxidative stress are associated differently with endothelial function and arterial stiffness in healthy subjects and in patients with atherosclerosis. [Published online ahead of print April 9 2008] *Scand J Clin Lab Invest*. 2008;68:1–8. Available at: http://www.ncbi.nlm.nih.gov/sites/entrez. Accessed 29 July 2008.

[30] Singh U, Jialal I. Oxidative stress and atherosclerosis. *Pathophysiology*. 2006;13:129–142.

[31] Booth AD, Wallace S, McEniery CM, et al. Inflammation and arterial stiffness in systemic vasculitis: a model of vascular inflammation. *Arthritis Rheum*. 2004;50:581–588.

[32] Couillard C, Ruel G, Archer WR, et al. Circulating levels of oxidative stress markers and endothelial adhesion molecules in men with abdominal obesity. *J Clin Endocrinol Metab*. 2005;90:6454–6459.

[33] Davì G, Guagnano MT, Ciabattoni G, et al. Platelet activation in obese women: role of inflammation and oxidant stress. *JAMA*. 2002;288:2008–2014.

[34] Vasdev S, Gill VD, Singal PK. Modulation of oxidative stressinduced changes in hypertension and atherosclerosis by antioxidants. *Exp Clin Cardol.* 2006;11:206–216.

[35] Flouris AD, Faught BE, Klentrou P. Cardiovascular disease risk in adolescent smokers: evidence of a smoker lifestyle. *J Child Health Care.* 2008;12:221–231.

[36] Neumann AI, Martins IS, Marcopito LF, Araujo EA. Dietary patterns associated with risk factors for cardiovascular disease in a Brazilian city. *Rev Panam Salud Publica.* 2007;22:329–339.

[37] Kamphuis MH, Geerlings MI, Tijhuis MA, et al. Physical inactivity, depression, and risk of cardiovascular mortality. *Med Sci Sports Exerc.* 2007;39:1693–1699.

[38] Gordon JL, Lavoie KL, Arsenault A, Ditto B, Bacon SL. Health behaviors and endothelial function. *J BehavMed.* 2008;31:5– 21.

[39] Wiersma JJ, Meuwese MC, van Miert JN, et al. Diabetes mellitus type 2 is associated with higher levels of myeloperoxidase. *Med Sci Monit.* 2008;14:CR 406–410.

[40] Valko M, Leibfritz D, Moncol J, Cronin MT, Mazur M, Telser J. Free radicals and antioxidants in normal physiological functions and human disease. *Int J Biochem Cell Biol.* 2007;39:44–84.

[41] Ceriello A, Motz E. Is oxidative stress the pathogenic mechanism underlying insulin resistance, diabetes, and cardiovascular disease? The common soil hypothesis revisited. *Arterioscler Thromb Vasc Biol.* 2004;24:816–823.

[42] Lavi S, Yang EH, Prasad A, et al. The interaction between coronary endothelial dysfunction, local oxidative stress, and endogenous nitric oxide in humans. *Hypertension.* 2008; 51:127–133.

[43] Kals J, Kampus P, Kals M, et al. Impact of oxidative stress on arterial elasticity in patients with atherosclerosis. *Am J Hypertens.* 2006;19:902–908.

[44] Hattori Y, MatsumuraM, Kasai K. Vascular smooth muscle cell activation by C-reactive protein. *Cardiovasc Res.* 2003;58:186–195.

[45] Yung LM, Leung FP, Yao X, Chen ZY, Huang Y. Reactive oxygen species in vascular wall. *Cardiovasc Hematol Disord Drug Targets.* 2006;6:1–19.

[46] Packard RR, Libby P. Inflammation in atherosclerosis: from vascular biology to biomarker discovery and risk prediction. *Clin Chem.* 2008;54:24–38.

[47] Libby P, Ridker PM, Maseri A. Inflammation and atherosclerosis. *Circulation*. 2002;105:1135–1143.

[48] Steinberg D, Witztum JL. Is the oxidative modification hypothesis relevant to human atherosclerosis? Do the antioxidant trials conducted to date refute the hypothesis? *Circulation*. 2002;105:2107–2111.

[49] Grattagliano I, Palmieri VO, Portincasa P, Moschetta A, Palasciano G. Oxidative stress-induced risk factors associated with the metabolic syndrome: a unifying hypothesis. *J Nutr Biochem*. 2008;19:491–504.

[50] Qamirani E, Ren Y, Kuo L, Hein TW. C-reactive protein inhibits endothelium-dependent NO-mediated dilation in coronary arterioles by activating p38 kinase and NAD(P)H oxidase. *Arterioscler Thromb Vasc Biol.* 2005;25:995–1001.

[51] Matsuura E, Kobayashi K, Tabuchi M, Lopez LR. Oxidative modification of low-density lipoprotein and immune regulation of atherosclerosis. *Prog Lipid Res*. 2006;45:466–486.

[52] Alexopoulos N, Vlachopoulos C, Aznaouridis K, et al. The acute effect of green tea consumption on endothelial function in healthy individuals. *Eur J Cardiovasc Prev Rehabil.* 2008;15:300–305.

[53] Shih PH, Yeh CT, Yen GC. Anthocyanins induce the activation of phase II enzymes through the antioxidant response element pathway against oxidative stress-induced apoptosis. *J Agric Food Chem.* 2007;55:9427–9435.

[54] Aviram M, Volkova N, Coleman R, et al. Pomegranate phenolics from the peels, arils, and flowers are antiatherogenic: studies in vivo in atherosclerotic apolipoprotein e-deficient (E 0) mice and in vitro in cultured macrophages and lipoproteins. *J Agric Food Chem.* 2008;56:1148–1157.

[55] de Nigris F, Balestrieri ML, Williams-Ignarro S, et al. The influence of pomegranate fruit extract in comparison to regular pomegranate juice and seed oil on nitric oxide and arterial function in obese Zucker rats. *Nitric Oxide*. 2007;17:50–54.

[56] Terao J, Kawai Y, Murota K. Vegetable flavonoids and cardiovascular disease. *Asia Pac J Clin Nutr*. 2008;17(Suppl 1):291–293.

[57] Spiller F, Alves MK, Vieira SM, et al. Anti-inflammatory effects of red pepper (*Capsicum baccatum*) on carrageenan- and antigen-induced inflammation. *J Pharm Pharmacol*. 2008;60: 473–478.

[58] Tribolo S, Lodi F, Connor C, et al. Comparative effects of quercetin and its predominant human metabolites on adhesion molecule expression in

activated human vascular endothelial cells. *Atherosclerosis.* 2008;197:50–56.

[59] Mertens-Talcott SU, Jilma-Stohlawetz P, Rios J, Hingorani L, Derendorf H. Absorption, metabolism, and antioxidant effects of pomegranate (*Punica granatum* L.) polyphenols after ingestion of a standardized extract in healthy human volunteers. *J Agric Food Chem.* 2006;54:8956–8961.

[60] Seeram NP, Aviram M, Zhang Y, et al. Comparison of antioxidant potency of commonly consumed polyphenol-rich beverages in the United States. *J Agric Food Chem.* 2008;56: 1415–1422.

[61] Gil MI, Tomás-Barberán FA, Hess-Pierce B, Holcroft DM, Kader AA. Antioxidant activity of pomegranate juice and its relationship with phenolic composition and processing. *J Agric Food Chem.* 2000;48:4581–4589.

[62] Azadzoi KM, Schulman RN, Aviram M, Siroky MB. Oxidative stress in arteriogenic erectile dysfunction: prophylactic role of antioxidants. *J Urol.* 2005;174:386–393.

[63] Rosenblat M, Aviram M. Antioxidative properties of pomegranate: in vitro studies. In: Seeram NP, Heber D, eds. *Pomegranates: Ancient Roots to Modern Medicine*. New York, NY: Taylor and Francis Group; 2006:31–43.

[64] Seeram NP, Lee R, Heber D. Bioavailability of ellagic acid in human plasma after consumption of ellagitannins from pomegranate (*Punica granatum* L.) juice. *Clin Chim Acta.* 2004;348:63–68.

[65] Seeram NP, Aviram M, Volkova N, Zhang Y, Henning SM, Nair M, Heber D. Dietary polyphenols derived from pomegranates are potent antioxidants: evaluation in various in vitro models of antioxidation. In: *228th National Meeting of the American Chemical Society*, American Chemical Society, Philadelphia, PA, 2004. Abstract AGFD44.

[66] Seeram NP, Henning SM, Zhang Y, Suchard M, Li Z, Heber D. Pomegranate juice ellagitannin metabolites are present in human plasma and some persist in urine for up to 48 hours. *J Nutr.* 2006;136:2481–2485.

[67] Cerdá B, Espín JC, Parra S,Martínez P, Tomás-Barberán FA. The potent in vitro antioxidant ellagitannins from pomegranate juice are metabolised into bioavailable but poor antioxidant hydroxy-6H-dibenzopyran-6-one derivatives by the colonic microflora of healthy humans. *Eur J Nutr.* 2004;43:205–220.

[68] Cerdá B, Soto C, Albaladejo MD, et al. Pomegranate juice supplementation in chronic obstructive pulmonary disease: a 5-week randomized, double-blind, placebo-controlled trial. *Eur J Clin Nutr.* 2006;60:245–253.
[69] Aviram M, Dornfeld L, Rosenblat M, et al. Pomegranate juice consumption reduces oxidative stress, atherogenic modifications of LDL, and platelet aggregation: studies in humans and in atherosclerotic apolipoprotein E-deficient mice. *Am J Clin Nutr.* 2000;71:1062–1076.
[70] Aviram M, Dornfeld L, Kaplan M, et al. Pomegranate juice flavonoids inhibit LDL oxidation and cardiovascular disease: studies in atherosclerotic mice and in humans. *Drugs Exp Clin Res.* 2002;28:49–62.
[71] Aviram M. Pomegranate juice as a major source for polyphenolic flavonoids and it is most potent antioxidant against LDL oxidation and atherosclerosis. *Free Radic Res.* 2002;36(Suppl 1):71–73.
[72] Kaplan M, Hayek T, Raz A, et al. Pomegranate juice supplementation to atherosclerotic mice reduces macrophage lipid peroxidation, cellular cholesterol accumulation and development of atherosclerosis. *J Nutr.* 2001;131:2082–2089.
[73] Napoli C, Ignarro LJ. Nitric oxide and atherosclerosis. *Nitric Oxide.* 2001;5:88–97.
[74] Ignarro LJ, Byrns RE, Sumi D, de Nigris F, Napoli C. Pomegranate juice protects nitric oxide against oxidative destruction and enhances the biological actions of nitric oxide. *Nitric Oxide.* 2006;15:93–102.
[75] Shukla M, Gupta K, Rasheed Z, Khan KA, Haqqi TM. Consumption of hydrolyzable tannins-rich pomegranate extract suppresses inflammation and joint damage in rheumatoid arthritis. *Nutrition.* 2008;24:733–743.
[76] Sartippour MR, Seeram NP, Rao JY, et al. Ellagitannin-rich pomegranate extract inhibits angiogenesis in prostate cancer in vitro and in vivo. *Int J Oncol.* 2008;32:475–480.
[77] Albrecht M, Jiang W, Kumi-Diaka J, et al. Pomegranate extracts potently suppress proliferation, xenograft growth, and invasion of human prostate cancer cells. *J. Med. Food.* 2004;7:274–283.
[78] Cerdá B, Cerón JJ, Tomás-Barberán FA, Espín JC. Repeated oral administration of high doses of the pomegranate ellagitannin punicalagin to rats for 37 days is not toxic. *J Agric Food Chem.* 2003;51:3493–3501.

[79] Esmaillzadeh A, Tahbaz F, Gaieni I, Alavi-Majd H, Azadbakht L. Concentrated pomegranate juice improves lipid profiles in diabetic patients with hyperlipidemia. *J Med Food*. 2004;7: 305–308.

[80] Rosenblat M, Hayek T, Aviram M. Anti-oxidative effects of pomegranate juice (PJ) consumption by diabetic patients on serum and on macrophages. *Atherosclerosis*. 2006;187:363– 371.

[81] Aviram M, Dornfeld L. Pomegranate juice consumption inhibits serum angiotensin converting enzyme activity and reduces systolic blood pressure. *Atherosclerosis*. 2001;158: 195–198.

[82] Tipoe GL, Leung TM, Hung MW, Fung ML. Green tea polyphenols as an anti-oxidant and anti-inflammatory agent for cardiovascular protection. *Cardiovasc Hematol Disord Drug Targets*. 2007;7:135–144.

[83] Misra A, Chattopadhyay R, Banerjee S, Chattopadhyay DJ Chatterjee IB. Black tea prevents cigarette smoke-induced oxidative damage of proteins in guinea pigs. *J Nutr*.2003;133:2622–2628.

[84] Hofmann T, Liegibel U,Winterhalter P, Bub A, Rechkemmer G, Pool-Zobel BL. Intervention with polyphenol-rich fruit juices results in an elevation of glutathione S-transferase P1 (hGSTP1) protein expression in human leucocytes of healthy volunteers. *Mol Nutr Food Res*. 2006;50:1191– 1200.

Chapter 7

ANTI-CANCER EFFECTS OF POMEGRANATES

ABSTRACT

Cancer is a disease whereby normal cells proliferate and divide at uncontrollable rates and often metastasize (or spread to other sites). Cancer is one of the leading causes of death in several countries. It represents the second leading cause of morbidity and mortality in the developed world second to diseases of the cardiovascular system. It can affect people of all ages, but is more likely in occur in middle and old age. Over 100 forms of cancers have been identified, most of which are described based on the organ of origin. Although several approaches have been developed for the treatment of cancers, not all have been successful. The rate of success is dependent on the type and location of the tumour, the stage of the disease, the person's age and general health. Surgery is often used to remove or excise a primary tumour, particularly those located around lymph nodes. Radiotherapy, involving high energy rays, is also used to directly target and inhibit the growth of cancer cells. Chemotherapeutics are used to induce cytotoxicity to tumour cells. However, as these strategies also target non-cancerous cells, there is a growing need to identify and develop natural products for the treatment of cancer with limited side effects. In-depth research into the anti-cancer activities of naturally occurring compounds present in pomegranates suggests provided renewed hope for natural alternative to cytotoxic chemotherapeutic agents that demonstrate significant cytotoxicity and adverse effects.

Introduction

Almost all tissues in the body can become malignant or cancerous. The most vulnerable sites include the skin, gastrointestinal system, the lungs and female breasts. Cancers can be classified into 3 types: Carcinomas are cancers which originate in the epithelial cells that form the skin and the linings of internal organs. Sarcomas are cancers which form in the connective tissue, such as muscle or bone. The third category is cancers of the blood (leukaemia) and the lymphatic system (lymphoma) [1-15]. Unlike benign tumors which cannot spread to other sites, a cancer, by definition, is malignant and capable of spreading further away from the site of origin. Cancers can spread to various parts of the body via the blood or lymphatic drainage. Most common is through the lymph nodes which drain tissues at the site where the tumour originated. For instance, breast cancer spreads to lymph nodes located in the axilla or armpit. Cancers which spread beyond the site of origin form tumors known as a metastasis. The cancer cells present in a metastasis are of the same type as in the primary tumour [16-20].

The aetiology of cancers remains unclear. Some cancers, namely melanoma, breast, ovary and colon cancer are hereditary. Others are associated with known risk factors. For example, cancers of the lungs, larynx, oesophagus, pancreas, bladder and kidney are linked to excessive tobacco smoking. A high fat diet may also contribute to the progression of cancers of the breast, colon, uterus, and prostate. Obesity is associated with increased rates of cancer of the prostate, pancreas, uterus, colon and ovary. Increased exposure to ultraviolet radiation can induce skin cancer. Chronic and excessive alcohol consumption may also cause cancers of the mouth, throat, oesophagus, larynx and the liver. The risk of cancer is also increased following exposure to several chemicals such as asbestos, nickel, cadmium, uranium and benzenes [21-25].

Clinical Applications of Pomegranates in Cancer Treatment

Pomegranate and Prostate Cancer

Initial studies by Albrecht et al. showed that supplementation with pomegranate juice and oil can inhibit proliferation and induced apoptosis in androgen dependent and independent prostate cancer cell lines without any cytotoxicity in normal primary prostate epithelial cells. Interestingly, pomegranate extracts also inhibited the growth of prostate cancer xenografts in nude mice. Recent reports suggests that these beneficial effects may be attributed to ellagitannins, which are abundant in pomegranates, and contribute enormously to the protective effects of pomegranates. Ellagic acid, caffeic acid, luteolin, and punicic acid, which are also present in pomegranate fruits, have also been shown to reduce the proliferation of invasiveness prostate cancer cells both *in vitro* and *in vivo*. It is likely that a combination of these important constituents may play a synergistic effect in inhibiting prostate cancer cell invasion across matrigel membranes *in vitro*. Pomegranates have also been shown to suppress of both androgen-synthesizing enzymes and androgen receptor expression. It was initially thought that pomegranate may exert its beneficial effect in prostate cancer cells by inhibiting the expression of genes involved in androgen synthesis. However, this mechanism remains unclear and further studies are needed to elucidate how the alteration of cell proliferation and apoptosis is related to the expression of androgen synthesizing enzymes and androgen receptor [26-31].

Constitutive nuclear factor kappa-light-chain-enhancer of activated B cells (NF-κB) signalling is almost always present in androgen-independent prostate cancer, and is used as a biomarker for tumour recurrence following surgery. Pomegranate extracts have been shown to inhibit NF-κB signalling, both in *in vitro* and *in vivo* prostate cancer models. Therefore, the induction of apoptosis in cancerous cells by pomegranate, *in vitro*, is likely to be attributed to its inhibitory effect on NF-κB activity. Several *in vivo* studies have used SCID mice implanted with LAPC4 prostate cancer cells, which are androgen dependent. These cancer cells cease growth on castration, and subsequently regrow after a latency of several weeks as androgen-independent tumors. In addition, LAPC4 cells exhibit constitutive NF-κB activity on emergence of the androgen independent state. Supplementation with pomegranate extracts derived from skins of fruit that it contained 37–40% punicalagins and 3.4% free ellagic acid significantly delayed growth compared with the castrate vehicle control group. Pomegranate extract also prevented the regrowth observed after castration and was associated with reduced NF-κB activity and serum NF-κB [31-35].

The molecular mechanisms associated with the anti-cancer activity of the pomegranate fruit have been previously investigated. Using MALDI-TOF Mass Spectrometry, the pomegranate fruit was shown to contain six major *anthocyanins* namely pelargonidin 3-glucoside, cyanidin 3-glucoside, delphinidin 3-glucoside, pelargonidin 3,5-diglucoside, cyaniding 3,5-diglucoside, and delphinidin 3,5-diglucoside; *ellagitannins* and hydrolysable *tannins*. These constituents can inhibit the growth and viability of prostate cancer cells through modulation of the cki-cyclin-cdk network, with up-regulation of p21 and p27 during G1-phase arrest, independent of p53. This correlated with down-regulation of the cyclins D1, D2, and E and cyclin-dependent kinases (cdk) −2, −4, and −6, operative in the G1 phase of the cell cycle. Supplementation with pomegranate extract (0.1% and 0.2%; wt/vol) in drinking water also attenuated tumour growth and decreased serum Prostate Specific Antigen (PSA) levels in athymic nude mice implanted with androgen-sensitive prostate cancer cells. The dose corresponds to a drink of 250 or 500 ml of pomegranate juice extracted from one or two fruits for a typical healthy individual weighing ~70 kg. Similarly, Seeram et al. showed a significant inhibition of LAPC-4 prostate cancer xenograft growth in the SCID mouse model fed an ellagitannin-enriched pomegranate extract diet orally [36-38].

In another study, a transgenic TRAMP mouse model received 0.1 and 0.2% pomegranate fruit extract, equivalent to 250 and 500 ml of pomegranate juice, in drinking water, starting at 6 weeks and examined at 12, 20 and 34 weeks of age. Prostate cancer in TRAMP mice progressed from precursor intraepithelial lesions, to invasive carcinoma that metastasizes to lymph nodes, liver, lungs, and occasionally to the bone similar to clinical prostate cancer. Remarkably, continuous supplementation of extract reduced tumour formation, decreased metastasis and conferred significant survival advantage, over water-fed controls. Tumour burden was also significantly lower in the extract-supplemented mice using magnetic resonance imaging. Additionally, the IGF-I/AKT/mTOR pathways were significantly inhibited in the prostate tissues and tumors of pomegranate treated animals. Koyama et al. showed that co-treatment of prostate cancer cells with pomegranate extract and IGFBP-3, a protein which is reduced during the progression of prostate cancer, can trigger apoptosis of tumour cells, increase JNK phosphorylation, suppress AKT/mTOR signalling and decrease IGF-1 mRNA levels, the latter of which is necessary for pomegranate-mediated apoptosis [39-40].

It has also been demonstrated that pomegranate juice can inhibit critical cellular processes associated with tumour invasion and metastasis, and production of pro-inflammatory cytokines (IL-6, -12p40, -1β and RANTES) which trigger tumour growth. Pomegranate juices can also upregulate the expression of genes involved in cellular adhesion, such as E-cadherin and intercellular adhesion molecule-1. Anti-invasive micro-RNAs (mi-RNAs) such as miR-335, miR-205, miR-200, and miR-126 are up-regulated, while proinvasive mi-RNAs such as miR-21 and miR-373 are down-regulated. Work by Pantuck et al. showed that pomegranate juice supplementation can prolong the PSA doubling time in patients suffering from the disease. In a small pilot study, patients with a detectable PSA of greater than 0.2 and less than 5 ng/mL were administered 8 ounces of pomegranate juice daily. No serious adverse events were reported upon completion of the study. Another study reported a 12% decrease in LnCaP prostate cancer cell proliferation, 17% increase in apoptosis, 23% increase in serum nitric oxide, and significant reductions in oxidative state and sensitivity to oxidation of serum lipids was observed, post treatment.

A recently single-arm phase II trial examined the effect of two doses of polyphenol-rich pomegranate fruit extract (POMx) in men with recurrent prostate cancer. The primary outcome was PSA doubling time. In this double-blind study patients with a rising PSA, without metastases, received 1 or 3 g of POMx. At completion of treatment (6 months), the median PSA doubling time lengthened from 11.9 months at baseline to 18.5 months, with no significant difference observed between dose groups. The results of this study remain unclear, warranting the need for further placebo-controlled studies. The anti-cancer effect of pomegranate is due to the accumulation of ellagitanins and their metabolites ellagic acid and urolithins in the human prostate. In one study with 63 patients with benign prostate hyperplasia (BPH) or prostate cancer, urolithin A glucuronide, urolithin B glucuronide, and dimethyl ellagic acid were present in a small number of prostates following pomegranate consumption, while no change in apoptotic enzyme, CDKN1A, MKi-67 or c-Myc were reported [40-41].

Pomegranate and Skin Cancer

Skin cancer represents the most common form of cancer in the United States, with the number of patients diagnosed exceeding three million skin cases annually. While the promotion of sun safety measures may partially reduce the number of skin cancer cases, there is an urgent need for the development of novel therapeutic agents for the prevention of skin cancer. A diet rich in phytochemicals may represent an alternative approach to treat reduce the high mortality rate associated with skin cancer

Pomegranate extracts have been shown to prevent effects of UV-A and UV-B radiation in primary human epidermal keratinocytes monolayer cell cultures. It is thought that pomegranate extract can inhibited UV-A mediated increase in the phosphorylation of ERK1/2 MAP Kinase, STAT-3 and the AKT/mTOR/p70S6Kinase pro-survival pathway and induced cell cycle arrest in the G-1 phase. UV-B induced phosphorylation of MAP Kinases (MAPKs) and activation and nuclear translocation of NF-κB was also inhibited by pomegranate extract treatment. POMx can also attenuate UV-B-induced lipid peroxidation, glutathione depletion, phosphorylation of MAPKs and c-Jun, and photo ageing in immortalized human HaCaT keratinocytes. As well, POMx has also been shown to protect skin fibroblasts from cell death following UV exposure, by reducing oxidative stress, inflammation, and the expression of the pro-apoptotic caspase-3, and an increase in G0/G1 phase associated with DNA repair. In the same study, the reduction in UV-induced oxidative stress and increase the intracellular antioxidant capacity correlated with the polyphenolic content of the pomegranate extract [42-44].

Pomegranate extracts have also been shown to protect against the formation of UV-B-induced cyclobutane pyrimidine dimers (CPD), and 8-dihydro-2′-deoxyguanosine (8-OHdG). This suggests that pomegranates can also augment the DNA repair system. Pomegranates can also inhibit UV-induced protein carbonyl formation and decreased the protein expression of proliferating cell nuclear antigen (PCNA). The consumption of pomegranates has also been shown to inhibit UV-B-induced edema, hyperplasia and leukocytic infiltration in the murine skin. A decrease in the expression of the inflammatory marker COX-2 and reduced activity the rate-limiting enzyme, ornithine decarboxylase (ODC), which is essential for the biosynthesis of polyamines, and required for the proliferation of malignant cancer cells has also been reported. It is well established that UV-B can induce DNA damage leading to phosphorylation of p53, leading to cell cycle arrest and allowing more time for the repair or elimination of damaged cells by apoptosis. A decrease in hydrogen peroxide generation and lipid peroxidation was observed in the extract-treated group in the 3-dimensional *in vitro* Epidermal model for skin cancer. In the same model, pomegranate treatment enhanced UV-B-mediated increases in p53 and p21 and decreased PCNA protein expression, and the number of CPDs and 8-OHdG in the mouse epidermis [45-47].

The polysaccharide fraction isolated from the rind of pomegranate possesses free radical scavenging, anti-glycation, and tyrosinase inhibition properties. Continuous oral administration of rind-derived pomegranate extract (100 mg/ml) to brown guinea pigs, for 35 days, were shown to inhibit UV-induced skin pigmentation and reduced the number of DOPA-positive melanocytes in the epidermis. Similarly, a double-blind, placebo-controlled human clinical trial showed that ellagic acid ingested orally had a skin whitening effect. This effect was further confirmed in another human trial where topical and oral administration of pomegranate attenuated the protective effect of sunscreens and afforded photo protection from UVB [48-51].

Pomegranate and Chemical Carcinogenesis

Pomegranates have also been shown to protect against chemical-induced carcinogenesis. In a 2- stage mouse skin tumorigenesis model for possible skin cancer chemopreventive efficacy, 7,12- dimethylbenzanthracene (DMBA) and Otetradecanoylphorbol 13-acetate (TPA) were used to initiate skin tumors in CD-1. Topical application of 5% pomegranate seed oil, prior to TPA yielded a 17% decrease in TPA stimulated ODC activity. As well, topical application of pomegranate fruit extract (2 mg/animal) prior to TPA, protected against TPA-mediated increase in skin edema and hyperplasia and epidermal ODC activity, reduced the protein expressions of ODC and COX-2, and inhibited TPA-induced phosphorylation of ERK1/2, p38, and JNK1/2 MAPKs and NF-κB activation in SKH-1 mice. Remarkably, only 30% of pomegranate treated mice developed tumors, compared to the control where 100% of the mice developed tumors at 16 weeks [52-53].

Pomegranate and Colon Cancer

Colon cancer is one of the most preventable forms of cancer, and dietary modifications are critical lifestyle measures that can reduce the risk of colon carcinogenesis. In particular, important polyphenols such as ellagitannins and urolithins have been shown to protect against the development of colon cancer due to their potent anti-inflammatory properties. One study reported a significant reduction in the expression of inflammatory markers such as PGE2, PAI-1 and IL-8, as well as other key regulators of cell migration and adhesion in colonic fibroblasts exposed to urolithins and ellagic acid, at doses achievable after oral consumption of pomegranates. This effect is likely to be due to the inhibition of activation of NF-κB and MAPKs, down-regulation of COX-2 and reduction of prostaglandin PGE2 production [54-44].

Several studies have been performed to determine the protective effects of pomegranates in colitis. In one study, intra-colonic administration of trinitrobenzene sulfonic acid (TNBS) produces inflammatory bowel disease in rats was used to closely mimic human colitis. Oral administration of ellagic acid (10 and 20 mg/kg) was able to attenuate the severity of intestinal injuries induced by TNBS in mice and reduced the size of intestinal lesions, enhanced the glandular architecture, reduced inflammatory cell infiltrate, and repressed COX-2 and iNOS pro-inflammatory proteins expression to basal levels. Bousetta et al. showed that the conjugated linolenic fatty acid, punicic acid, a major fatty acid present in pomegranate seed oil displayed a strong inhibitory effect on TNFα-induced oxidative stress by neutrophils, by inhibiting the phosphorylation at Ser345, and p38MAPKinase [56-60].

Pomegranate juice derived ellagitannins and their intestinal bacterial metabolites urolithins have also been shown to be protective in several *in vitro* models. Both ellagitannins and urolithins inhibited CYP1 activity, suppressed cell proliferation and decreased clonogenic efficiency of HT-29 colon cancer cells. Inhibition of cell proliferation was mediated through cell cycle arrest in the G0/G1 and G2/M stages of the cell cycle followed by induction of apoptosis. Adams et al. showed that pomegranate juice significantly suppressed TNFα-induced COX-2 protein expression, AKT activation and NF-κB binding activity in these cells. Interestingly, ellagic acid alone was unable to suppress NF-κB binding activity. This suggests that other polyphenols such as anthocyanins and flavonols present in pomegranates may account for the enhanced anti-proliferative activity. Evidence for this comes from the work by Seeram et al. who showed that pomegranate juice possesses greater antioxidant activity than punicalagin and ellagic acid [61-69].

Pomegranate and Lung Cancer

Inflammation appears to play a causal role in the development of lung cancer. Inflammation promotes the recruitment of macrophages, slows the clearance of neutrophils and stimulates free radical production. It is therefore not surprising that pomegranates have been suggested to play a potential therapeutic role in the treatment of lung cancer. Pomegranate peel extracts have been shown to reduce neutrophil free radical production, *in vitro,* and on lipopolysaccharide-induced lung inflammation, in mice. However, the extract had no effect on superoxide anion generation *in vitro*, suggesting that it does not directly inhibit NADPH oxidase activity, or scavenge superoxide anions [69].

The effect of oral consumption of a human achievable dose of pomegranate fruit extract on mice implanted with human lung carcinoma A549 xenografts has also been previously investigated. Pomegranate treatment selectively decreased the viability of A549 cells, but had minimal effect on normal bronchial cells *in vitro*. In particular, pomegranate treatment arrested cells in G0-G1 phase of the cell cycle with induction of p21 and p27, decrease in cyclins D1, D2 and E and cdks −2, −4 and −6 protein expressions, and inhibited MAPKinase phosphorylation, and reduced the protein expression of proliferation markers Ki-67 and PCNA [70].

Another study showed that tumour growth can be significantly reduced following oral administration of pomegranate fruit extract 0.1% and 0.2% (wt/vol) to athymic nude mice implanted with A549 cells. Supplementation with 0.2% pomegranate fruit extract (w/v) was able to reduce the growth, progression and angiogenesis of tumors in two mouse lung tumour models where cancer was induced by benzo(a)pyrene and N-nitroso-trischloroethylurea in A/J mice. Consistent with previous studies, tumour studies reported similar inhibition of MAPKs, PI3K/AKT and NF-κB signalling pathways in the extract treated mice [71].

Pomegranate and Breast Cancer

The proliferation of breast cancer cells and the growth of oestrogen-responsive tumors are enhanced by oestrogen. Several pomegranate-derived compounds have been shown to inhibit the activity of the enzyme aromatase, which stimulates oestrogen production. These compounds include ellagic acid, gallagic acid, and urolithins A and B (and their acetylated, methylated, and sulfated analogues). However, Urolithin B has been shown to be the most effective in inhibiting testosterone-induced breast cancer cell proliferation and inhibiting aromatase activity [72-75].

Pomegranate juice has been shown to inhibit endogenous active oestrogen biosynthesis and inhibited the catalytic activity of the steroid-converting enzyme, 17-beta-hydroxysteroid dehydrogenase-1. Pomegranate juice showed anti-proliferative activity in both oestrogen sensitive MCF-7 and oestrogen resistant MB-MDA-231 cells. Similarly, pomegranate juice sufficiently inhibited DMBA-induced cancerous lesion formation in murine mammary glands. Punicic acid, an important omega-5 long chain polyunsaturated fatty acid present in the pomegranate seed oil inhibited proliferation and induced apoptosis in oestrogen sensitive and insensitive breast cancer cell lines, dependent on lipid peroxidation and the PKC pathway. Oestrogen receptor activity is modulated by pomegranate seed linolenic acid isomers in a concentration dependent manner. Pomegranate extract in combination with genistein was more effective than the individual treatment in inhibiting growth of breast cancer cells and induction of apoptosis. The decrease in proliferation, invasion, and motility in aggressive breast cancer phenotypes with pomegranate fruit extract treatment is likely to be attributed to the suppression of NF-κB gene expression and a decrease in RhoC and RhoA protein expression [76-77].

Pomegranate juice has also been shown to reduce inflammation and angiogenesis in the conditioned media of MCF-7 or MDA-MB-231 human breast cancer cells. These observations were accompanied by reduced expression of VEGF and up-regulation of migration inhibitory factor. The significant reduction in new blood vessel formation in the chicken chorioallantoic membrane model further demonstrates the potent anti-angiogenic properties of pomegranates [78-79].

Pomegranate and Leukemia

Recent studies have shown that pomegranates may also be useful against leukaemia. The rind of pomegranate fruit contains the polysaccharide PSP001, which can inhibit the growth of leukaemia cell lines. Pomegranate juice can also stimulate apoptosis of lymphoid and myeloid leukaemia cell lines. There is also evidence that pomegranate fruit extract can promote differentiation in human leukaemia cells although this is yet to be validated [80-83].

Future Prospects and Conclusion

Cancer remains the leading cause of human mortality. The potential beneficial effects of diverse dietary phytochemical agents is of major interest in the biological activities of pomegranate-derived products, particularly to their anti-cancer properties (Figure 1). Pomegranate juice has shown promise against prostate and other others both *in vitro*, *in vivo* and in a selection of human clinical trials. A major limitation in clinical studies investigating the preventive effect of pomegranate is to show the absence or reduced incidence of a specific disease end point. In addition, new biomarkers accurately analyse the long term disease prevention. No major adverse health effects have been reported following consumption of pomegranate juice. Finally, the combinatory effect of pomegranate with other compounds remains to be investigated. Whether pomegranates can amplify the chemoprotective effects of other agents via an additive but also synergistic or even antagonistic effect is crucial for developing effective treatment regimen in cancer.

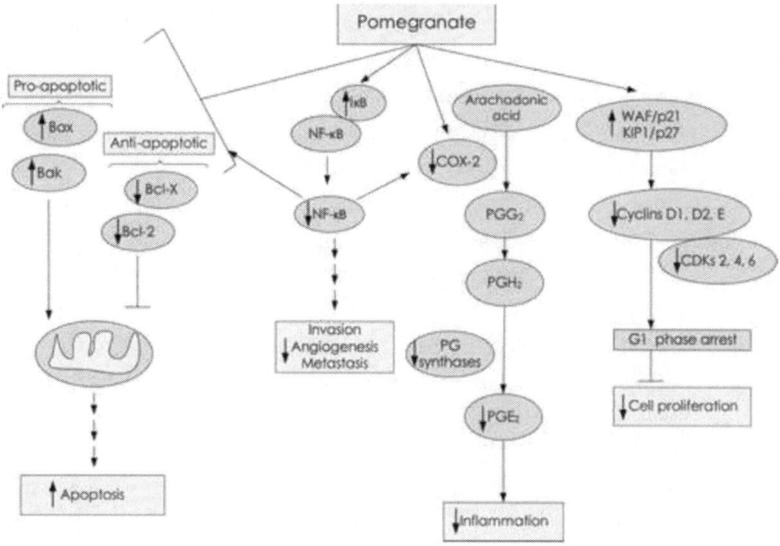

Figure 1. Schematic Representation of the molecular and cellular target of pomegranate constituents in Cancer.

REFERENCES

[1] Mukhtar H, Ahmad N. Cancer chemoprevention: future holds in multiple agents. *Toxicol. Appl. Pharmacol.* 1999; 158(3):207–10. [PubMed: 10438653]

[2] Syed DN, Afaq F, Mukhtar H. Pomegranate derived products for cancer chemoprevention. *Semin. Cancer Biol.* 2007; 17(5):377–85. [PubMed: 17613245]

[3] de Kok TM, de Waard P, Wilms LC, van Breda SG. Antioxidative and antigenotoxic properties of vegetables and dietary phytochemicals: the value of genomics biomarkers in molecular epidemiology. *Mol. Nutr. Food Res.* 2010; 54(2):208–17.

[4] Schwartz E, Tzulker R, Glazer I, Bar-Ya'akov I, Wiesman Z, Tripler E, Bar-Ilan I, Fromm H, Borochov-Neori H, Holland D, Amir R. Environmental conditions affect the color, taste, and antioxidant capacity

of 11 pomegranate accessions' fruits. *J. Agr. Food Chem.* 2009; 57(19):9197–209. [PubMed: 19725542]

[5] Aviram M, Kaplan M, Rosenblat M, Fuhrman B. Dietary antioxidants and paraoxonases against LDL oxidation and atherosclerosis development. *Handbook of Exp. Pharmacol.* 2005; (170): 263–300.

[6] Kaufman M, Wiesman Z. Pomegranate oil analysis with emphasis on MALDI-TOF/MS triacylglycerol fingerprinting. *J. Agr. Food Chem.* 2007; 55(25):10405–13. [PubMed: 18004807]

[7] Gil MI, Tomas-Barberan FA, Hess-Pierce B, Holcroft DM, Kader AA. Antioxidant activity of pomegranate juice and its relationship with phenolic composition and processing. *J. Agr. Food Chem.* 2000; 48(10):4581–9. [PubMed: 11052704]

[8] Guo S, Deng Q, Xiao J, Xie B, Sun Z. Evaluation of antioxidant activity and preventing DNA damage effect of pomegranate extracts by chemiluminescence method. *J. Agr. Food Chem.* 2007; 55(8):3134–40. [PubMed: 17381116]

[9] Rababah TM, Banat F, Rababah A, Ereifej K, Yang W. Optimization of extraction conditions of total phenolics, antioxidant activities, and anthocyanin of oregano, thyme, terebinth, and pomegranate. *J. Food Sci.* 2010; 75(7):C626–32. [PubMed: 21535529]

[10] Qu W, Breksa AP Iii, Pan Z, Ma H, McHugh TH. Storage stability of sterilized liquid extracts from pomegranate peel. *J. Food Sci.* 2012; 77(7):C765–72. [PubMed: 22757697]

[11] Mirdehghan SH, Rahemi M, Serrano M, Guillen F, Martinez-Romero D, Valero D. The application of polyamines by pressure or immersion as a tool to maintain functional properties in stored pomegranate arils. *J. Agr. Food Chem.* 2007; 55(3):755–60. [PubMed: 17263471]

[12] Fischer UA, Jaksch AV, Carle R, Kammerer DR. Determination of lignans in edible and nonedible parts of pomegranate (Punica granatum L.) and products derived therefrom, particularly focusing on the quantitation of isolariciresinol using HPLC-DAD-ESI/MSn. *J. Agr. Food Chem.* 2012; 60(1):283–92. [PubMed: 22136560]

[13] Malik A, Afaq F, Sarfaraz S, Adhami VM, Syed DN, Mukhtar H. Pomegranate fruit juice for chemoprevention and chemotherapy of prostate cancer. *Proc Natl Acad Sci U S A.* 2005;102(41):14813–8. [PubMed: 16192356]

[14] Khan N, Afaq F, Kweon MH, Kim K, Mukhtar H. Oral consumption of pomegranate fruit extract inhibits growth and progression of primary

lung tumors in mice. *Cancer Res.* 2007; 67(7):3475–82. [PubMed: 17389758]

[15] Perez-Vicente A, Gil-Izquierdo A, Garcia-Viguera C. *In vitro* gastrointestinal digestion study of pomegranate juice phenolic compounds, anthocyanins, and vitamin C. *J. Agr. Food Chem.* 2002; 50(8):2308–12. [PubMed: 11929289]

[16] Cerda B, Llorach R, Ceron JJ, Espin JC, Tomas-Barberan FA. Evaluation of the bioavailability and metabolism in the rat of punicalagin, an antioxidant polyphenol from pomegranate juice. *Eu. J. Nutr.* 2003; 42(1):18–28.

[17] Cerda B, Espin JC, Parra S, Martinez P, Tomas-Barberan FA. The potent *in vitro* antioxidant ellagitannins from pomegranate juice are metabolised into bioavailable but poor antioxidant hydroxy-6H-dibenzopyran-6-one derivatives by the colonic microflora of healthy humans. *Eu. J. Nutr.* 2004; 43(4):205–20.

[18] Cerda B, Tomas-Barberan FA, Espin JC. Metabolism of antioxidant and chemopreventive ellagitannins from strawberries, raspberries, walnuts, and oak-aged wine in humans: identification of biomarkers and individual variability. *J. Agr. Food Chem.* 2005; 53(2):227–35. [PubMed: 15656654]

[19] Espin JC, Gonzalez-Barrio R, Cerda B, Lopez-Bote C, Rey AI, Tomas-Barberan FA. Iberian pig as a model to clarify obscure points in the bioavailability and metabolism of ellagitannins in humans. *J. Agr. Food Chem.* 2007; 55(25):10476–85. [PubMed: 17990850]

[20] Neyrinck AM, Van Hee VF, Bindels LB, De Backer F, Cani PD, Delzenne NM. Polyphenol-rich extract of pomegranate peel alleviates tissue inflammation and hypercholesterolaemia in high-fat diet-induced obese mice: potential implication of the gut microbiota. *Br. J. Nutr.* 2012:1–8.

[21] Seeram NP, Lee R, Heber D. Bioavailability of ellagic acid in human plasma after consumption of ellagitannins from pomegranate (Punica granatum L.) juice. *Clinica Chimica Acta: Int. J. Clin. Chem.* 2004; 348(1-2):63–8.

[22] Mertens-Talcott SU, Jilma-Stohlawetz P, Rios J, Hingorani L, Derendorf H. Absorption, metabolism, and antioxidant effects of pomegranate (Punica granatum l.) polyphenols after ingestion of a standardized extract in healthy human volunteers. *J. Agr. Food Chem.* 2006; 54(23):8956–61. [PubMed: 17090147]

[23] Seeram NP, Henning SM, Zhang Y, Suchard M, Li Z, Heber D. Pomegranate juice ellagitannin metabolites are present in human plasma and some persist in urine for up to 48 hours. *J. Nutr.* 2006; 136(10):2481–5. [PubMed: 16988113]

[24] Bialonska D, Kasimsetty SG, Khan SI, Ferreira D. Urolithins, intestinal microbial metabolites of Pomegranate ellagitannins, exhibit potent antioxidant activity in a cell-based assay. *J. Agr. Food Chem.* 2009; 57(21):10181–6. [PubMed: 19824638]

[25] Seeram NP, Zhang Y, McKeever R, Henning SM, Lee RP, Suchard MA, Li Z, Chen S, Thames G, Zerlin A, Nguyen M, Wang D, Dreher M, Heber D. Pomegranate juice and extracts provide similar levels of plasma and urinary ellagitannin metabolites in human subjects. *J. Med. Food.* 2008; 11(2):390–4. [PubMed: 18598186]

[26] Lansky EP, Jiang W, Mo H, Bravo L, Froom P, Yu W, Harris NM, Neeman I, Campbell MJ. Possible synergistic prostate cancer suppression by anatomically discrete pomegranate fractions. *Invest. New Drugs.* 2005; 23(1):11–20. [PubMed: 15528976]

[27] Albrecht M, Jiang W, Kumi-Diaka J, Lansky EP, Gommersall LM, Patel A, Mansel RE, Neeman I, Geldof AA, Campbell MJ. Pomegranate extracts potently suppress proliferation, xenograft growth, and invasion of human prostate cancer cells. *J. Med. Food.* 2004; 7(3):274–83. [PubMed: 15383219]

[28] Lansky EP, Harrison G, Froom P, Jiang WG. Pomegranate (Punica granatum) pure chemicals show possible synergistic inhibition of human PC-3 prostate cancer cell invasion across Matrigel. *Invest. new drugs.* 2005; 23(2):121–2. [PubMed: 15744587]

[29] Hong MY, Seeram NP, Heber D. Pomegranate polyphenols down-regulate expression of androgen-synthesizing genes in human prostate cancer cells overexpressing the androgen receptor. *J. Nutr. Biochem.* 2008; 19(12):848–55. [PubMed: 18479901]

[30] Rettig MB, Heber D, An J, Seeram NP, Rao JY, Liu H, Klatte T, Belldegrun A, Moro A, Henning SM, Mo D, Aronson WJ, Pantuck A. Pomegranate extract inhibits androgenindependent prostate cancer growth through a nuclear factor-kappaB-dependent mechanism. *Mol. Cancer Ther.* 2008; 7(9):2662–71. [PubMed: 18790748]

[31] Afaq F, Saleem M, Krueger CG, Reed JD, Mukhtar H. Anthocyanin- and hydrolyzable tanninrich pomegranate fruit extract modulates MAPK and NF-kappaB pathways and inhibits skin tumorigenesis in CD-1 mice. *Int. J. Cancer. J. Int. Du Cancer.* 2005; 113(3):423–33.

[32] Seeram NP, Aronson WJ, Zhang Y, Henning SM, Moro A, Lee RP, Sartippour M, Harris DM, Rettig M, Suchard MA, Pantuck AJ, Belldegrun A, Heber D. Pomegranate ellagitannin-derived metabolites inhibit prostate cancer growth and localize to the mouse prostate gland. *J. Agr. Food Chem.* 2007; 55(19):7732–7. [PubMed: 17722872]

[33] Adhami VM, Siddiqui IA, Syed DN, Lall RK, Mukhtar H. Oral infusion of pomegranate fruit extract inhibits prostate carcinogenesis in the TRAMP model. *Carcinogenesis.* 2012; 33(3):644– 51. [PubMed: 22198212]

[34] Koyama S, Cobb LJ, Mehta HH, Seeram NP, Heber D, Pantuck AJ, Cohen P. Pomegranate extract induces apoptosis in human prostate cancer cells by modulation of the IGF-IGFBP axis. *Growth Hormone & IGF Res.* 2010; 20(1):55–62.

[35] Seeram NP, Adams LS, Henning SM, Niu Y, Zhang Y, Nair MG, Heber D. *In vitro* antiproliferative, apoptotic and antioxidant activities of punicalagin, ellagic acid and a total pomegranate tannin extract are enhanced in combination with other polyphenols as found in pomegranate juice. *J. Nutr. Biochem.* 2005; 16(6):360–7. [PubMed: 15936648]

[36] Wang L, Alcon A, Yuan H, Ho J, Li QJ, Martins-Green M. Cellular and molecular mechanisms of pomegranate juice-induced anti-metastatic effect on prostate cancer cells. *Integr. Biol.* 2011; 3(7):742–54.

[37] Pantuck AJ, Leppert JT, Zomorodian N, Aronson W, Hong J, Barnard RJ, Seeram N, Liker H, Wang H, Elashoff R, Heber D, Aviram M, Ignarro L, Belldegrun A. Phase II study of pomegranate juice for men with rising prostate-specific antigen following surgery or radiation for prostate cancer. *Clin. Cancer Res.* 2006; 12(13):4018–26. [PubMed: 16818701]

[38] Paller CJ, Ye X, Wozniak PJ, Gillespie BK, Sieber PR, Greengold RH, Stockton BR, Hertzman BL, Efros MD, Roper RP, Liker HR, Carducci MA. A randomized phase II study of pomegranate extract for men with rising PSA following initial therapy for localized prostate cancer. *Prostate Cancer And Prostatic Diseases.* 2012

[39] Gonzalez-Sarrias A, Gimenez-Bastida JA, Garcia-Conesa MT, Gomez-Sanchez MB, Garcia- Talavera NV, Gil-Izquierdo A, Sanchez-Alvarez C, Fontana-Compiano LO, Morga-Egea JP, Pastor-Quirante FA, Martinez-Diaz F, Tomas-Barberan FA, Espin JC. Occurrence of urolithins, gut microbiota ellagic acid metabolites and proliferation markers expression response in the human prostate gland upon

consumption of walnuts and pomegranate juice. *Mol. Nutr. Food Res.* 2010; 54(3):311–22. [PubMed: 19885850]

[40] Kasimsetty SG, Bialonska D, Reddy MK, Thornton C, Willett KL, Ferreira D. Effects of pomegranate chemical constituents/intestinal microbial metabolites on CYP1B1 in 22Rv1 prostate cancer cells. *J. Agr. Food Chem.* 2009; 57(22):10636–44. [PubMed: 19919114]

[41] Faria A, Monteiro R, Azevedo I, Calhau C. Pomegranate juice effects on cytochrome P450S expression: *in vivo* studies. *J. Med. Food.* 2007; 10(4):643–9. [PubMed: 18158835]

[42] Syed DN, Malik A, Hadi N, Sarfaraz S, Afaq F, Mukhtar H. Photochemopreventive effect of pomegranate fruit extract on UVA-mediated activation of cellular pathways in normal human epidermal keratinocytes. *Photochem. Photobiol.* 2006; 82(2):398–405. [PubMed: 16613491]

[43] Afaq F, Malik A, Syed D, Maes D, Matsui MS, Mukhtar H. Pomegranate fruit extract modulates UV-B-mediated phosphorylation of mitogen-activated protein kinases and activation of nuclear factor kappa B in normal human epidermal keratinocytes paragraph sign. *Photochem. Photobiol.* 2005; 81(1):38–45. [PubMed: 15493960]

[44] Zaid MA, Afaq F, Syed DN, Dreher M, Mukhtar H. Inhibition of UVB-mediated oxidative stress and markers of photoaging in immortalized HaCaT keratinocytes by pomegranate polyphenol extract POMx. *Photochem. Photobiol.* 2007; 83(4):882–8. [PubMed: 17645659]

[45] Pacheco-Palencia LA, Noratto G, Hingorani L, Talcott ST, Mertens-Talcott SU. Protective effects of standardized pomegranate (Punica granatum L.) polyphenolic extract in ultravioletirradiated human skin fibroblasts. *J. Agr. Food Chem.* 2008; 56(18):8434–41. [PubMed: 18717570]

[46] Afaq F, Zaid MA, Khan N, Dreher M, Mukhtar H. Protective effect of pomegranate-derived products on UVB-mediated damage in human reconstituted skin. *Exp. Dermatol.* 2009; 18(6): 553–61. [PubMed: 19320737]

[47] Afaq F, Khan N, Syed DN, Mukhtar H. Oral feeding of pomegranate fruit extract inhibits early biomarkers of UVB radiation-induced carcinogenesis in SKH-1 hairless mouse epidermis. *Photochem. Photobiol.* 2010; 86(6):1318–26. [PubMed: 20946358]

[48] Khan N, Syed DN, Pal HC, Mukhtar H, Afaq F. Pomegranate Fruit Extract Inhibits UVB induced Inflammation and Proliferation by

Modulating NF-kappaB and MAPK Signaling Pathways in Mouse Skin(dagger). *Photochem. Photobiol.* 2011

[49] Rout S, Banerjee R. Free radical scavenging, anti-glycation and tyrosinase inhibition properties of a polysaccharide fraction isolated from the rind from Punica granatum. *Bioresource Technol.* 2007; 98(16):3159–63.

[50] Yoshimura M, Watanabe Y, Kasai K, Yamakoshi J, Koga T. Inhibitory effect of an ellagic acidrich pomegranate extract on tyrosinase activity and ultraviolet-induced pigmentation. *Biosci. Biotechnol. Biochem.* 2005; 69(12):2368–73. [PubMed: 16377895]

[51] Kasai K, Yoshimura M, Koga T, Arii M, Kawasaki S. Effects of oral administration of ellagic acid-rich pomegranate extract on ultraviolet-induced pigmentation in the human skin. J. *Nutr. Sci. Vitaminol.* 2006; 52(5):383–8. [PubMed: 17190110]

[52] Hora JJ, Maydew ER, Lansky EP, Dwivedi C. Chemopreventive effects of pomegranate seed oil on skin tumor development in CD1 mice. *J. Med. Food.* 2003; 6(3):157–61. [PubMed: 14585180]

[53] George J, Singh M, Srivastava AK, Bhui K, Shukla Y. Synergistic growth inhibition of mouse skin tumors by pomegranate fruit extract and diallyl sulfide: evidence for inhibition of activated MAPKs/NF-kappaB and reduced cell proliferation. *Food Chem. Toxicol.* 2011; 49(7):1511–20. [PubMed: 21443920]

[54] Aslam MN, Lansky EP, Varani J. Pomegranate as a cosmeceutical source: pomegranate fractions promote proliferation and procollagen synthesis and inhibit matrix metalloproteinase-1 production in human skin cells. *J. Ethnopharmacol.* 2006; 103(3):311–8. [PubMed: 16221534]

[55] Murthy KN, Reddy VK, Veigas JM, Murthy UD. Study on wound healing activity of Punica granatum peel. *J. Med. Food.* 2004; 7(2):256–9. [PubMed: 15298776]

[56] Hayouni EA, Miled K, Boubaker S, Bellasfar Z, Abedrabba M, Iwaski H, Oku H, Matsui T, Limam F, Hamdi M. Hydroalcoholic extract based-ointment from Punica granatum L. peels with enhanced *in vivo* healing potential on dermal wounds. *Phytomedicine.* 2011; 18(11):976–84. [PubMed: 21466954]

[57] Gimenez-Bastida JA, Larrosa M, Gonzalez-Sarrias A, Tomas-Barberan F, Espin JC, Garcia- Conesa MT. Intestinal Ellagitannin Metabolites Ameliorate Cytokine-Induced Inflammation and Associated Molecular Markers in Human Colon Fibroblasts. *J. Agr. Food Chem.* 2012

[58] Gonzalez-Sarrias A, Larrosa M, Tomas-Barberan FA, Dolara P, Espin JC. NF-kappaB-dependent anti-inflammatory activity of urolithins, gut microbiota ellagic acid-derived metabolites, in human colonic fibroblasts. *Br. J. Nutr.* 2010; 104(4):503–12. [PubMed: 20338073]

[59] Rosillo MA, Sanchez-Hidalgo M, Cardeno A, de la Lastra CA. Protective effect of ellagic acid, a natural polyphenolic compound, in a murine model of Crohn's disease. *Biochem. Pharmacol.* 2011; 82(7):737–45. [PubMed: 21763290]

[60] Boussetta T, Raad H, Letteron P, Gougerot-Pocidalo MA, Marie JC, Driss F, El-Benna J. Punicic acid a conjugated linolenic acid inhibits TNFalpha-induced neutrophil hyper-activation and protects from experimental colon inflammation in rats. *PloS one*. 2009; 4(7):e6458. [PubMed: 19649246]

[61] Larrosa M, Gonzalez-Sarrias A, Yanez-Gascon MJ, Selma MV, Azorin-Ortuno M, Toti S, Tomas-Barberan F, Dolara P, Espin JC. Anti-inflammatory properties of a pomegranate extract and its metabolite urolithin-A in a colitis rat model and the effect of colon inflammation on phenolic metabolism. *J. Nutr. Biochem.* 2010; 21(8):717–25. [PubMed: 19616930]

[62] Ogawa Y, Kanatsu K, Iino T, Kato S, Jeong YI, Shibata N, Takada K, Takeuchi K. Protection against dextran sulfate sodium-induced colitis by microspheres of ellagic acid in rats. *Life Sci.* 2002; 71(7):827–39. [PubMed: 12074942]

[63] Singh K, Jaggi AS, Singh N. Exploring the ameliorative potential of Punica granatum in dextran sulfate sodium induced ulcerative colitis in mice. *Phytotherapy Res.* 2009; 23(11):1565–74.

[64] Kasimsetty SG, Bialonska D, Reddy MK, Ma G, Khan SI, Ferreira D. Colon cancer chemopreventive activities of pomegranate ellagitannins and urolithins. *J. Agr. Food Chem.* 2010; 58(4):2180–7. [PubMed: 20112993]

[65] Adams LS, Seeram NP, Aggarwal BB, Takada Y, Sand D, Heber D. Pomegranate juice, total pomegranate ellagitannins, and punicalagin suppress inflammatory cell signaling in colon cancer cells. *J. Agr. Food Chem.* 2006; 54(3):980–5. [PubMed: 16448212]

[66] Larrosa M, Tomas-Barberan FA, Espin JC. The dietary hydrolysable tannin punicalagin releases ellagic acid that induces apoptosis in human colon adenocarcinoma Caco-2 cells by using the mitochondrial pathway. *J. Nutr. Biochem.* 2006; 17(9):611–25. [PubMed: 16426830]

[67] Sharma M, Li L, Celver J, Killian C, Kovoor A, Seeram NP. Effects of fruit ellagitannin extracts, ellagic acid, and their colonic metabolite, urolithin A, on Wnt signaling. *J. Agr. Food Chem.* 2010; 58(7):3965–9. [PubMed: 20014760]

[68] Kohno H, Suzuki R, Yasui Y, Hosokawa M, Miyashita K, Tanaka T. Pomegranate seed oil rich in conjugated linolenic acid suppresses chemically induced colon carcinogenesis in rats. *Cancer Sci.* 2004; 95(6):481–6. [PubMed: 15182427]

[69] Cho WC, Kwan CK, Yau S, So PP, Poon PC, Au JS. The role of inflammation in the pathogenesis of lung cancer. *Exp. Opin. Therap. Targets.* 2011; 15(9):1127–37.

Bachoual R, Talmoudi W, Boussetta T, Braut F, El-Benna J. An aqueous pomegranate peel extract inhibits neutrophil myeloperoxidase *in vitro* and attenuates lung inflammation in mice. *Food Chem. Toxicol.* 2011; 49(6):1224–8. [PubMed: 21376769]

[70] Khan N, Hadi N, Afaq F, Syed DN, Kweon MH, Mukhtar H. Pomegranate fruit extract inhibits prosurvival pathways in human A549 lung carcinoma cells and tumor growth in athymic nude mice. *Carcinogenesis.* 2007; 28(1):163–73. [PubMed: 16920736]

[71] Adams LS, Zhang Y, Seeram NP, Heber D, Chen S. Pomegranate ellagitannin-derived compounds exhibit antiproliferative and antiaromatase activity in breast cancer cells *in vitro*. *Cancer Prev. Res.* 2010; 3(1):108–13.

[72] Kim ND, Mehta R, Yu W, Neeman I, Livney T, Amichay A, Poirier D, Nicholls P, Kirby A, Jiang W, Mansel R, Ramachandran C, Rabi T, Kaplan B, Lansky E. Chemo-preventive and adjuvant therapeutic potential of pomegranate (Punica granatum) for human breast cancer. *Breast Cancer Res. Treatment.* 2002; 71(3):203–17.

[73] Grossmann ME, Mizuno NK, Schuster T, Cleary MP. Punicic acid is an omega-5 fatty acid capable of inhibiting breast cancer proliferation. *Int. J. Oncol.* 2010; 36(2):421–6. [PubMed: 20043077]

[74] Tran HN, Bae SY, Song BH, Lee BH, Bae YS, Kim YH, Lansky EP, Newman RA. Pomegranate (Punica granatum) seed linolenic acid isomers: concentration-dependent modulation of estrogen receptor activity. *Endocrine Res.* 2010; 35(1):1–16. [PubMed: 20136514]

[75] Mehta R, Lansky EP. Breast cancer chemopreventive properties of pomegranate (Punica granatum) fruit extracts in a mouse mammary organ culture. *Eu. J. Cancer Prev.* 2004; 13(4): 345–8.

[76] Jeune MA, Kumi-Diaka J, Brown J. Anticancer activities of pomegranate extracts and genistein in human breast cancer cells. *J. Med. Food.* 2005; 8(4):469–75. [PubMed: 16379557]

[77] Khan GN, Gorin MA, Rosenthal D, Pan Q, Bao LW, Wu ZF, Newman RA, Pawlus AD, Yang P, Lansky EP, Merajver SD. Pomegranate fruit extract impairs invasion and motility in human breast cancer. *Integrat. Cancer Therapies.* 2009; 8(3):242–53.

[78] Toi M, Bando H, Ramachandran C, Melnick SJ, Imai A, Fife RS, Carr RE, Oikawa T, Lansky EP. Preliminary studies on the anti-angiogenic potential of pomegranate fractions *in vitro* and *in vivo*. *Angiogenesis.* 2003; 6(2):121–8. [PubMed: 14739618]

[79] Joseph MM, Aravind SR, Varghese S, Mini S, Sreelekha TT. Evaluation of antioxidant, antitumor and immunomodulatory properties of polysaccharide isolated from fruit rind of Punica granatum. *Mol. Med. Rep.* 2012; 5(2):489–96. [PubMed: 22012001]

[80] Dahlawi H, Jordan-Mahy N, Clench MR, Le Maitre CL. Bioactive actions of pomegranate fruit extracts on leukemia cell lines *in vitro* hold promise for new therapeutic agents for leukemia. *Nutr. Cancer.* 2012; 64(1):100–10. [PubMed: 22098126]

[81] Li Z, Percival SS, Bonard S, Gu L. Fabrication of nanoparticles using partially purified pomegranate ellagitannins and gelatin and their apoptotic effects. *Mol. Nutr. Food Res.* 2011; 55(7):1096–103. [PubMed: 21374799]

[82] Kawaii S, Lansky EP. Differentiation-promoting activity of pomegranate (Punica granatum) fruit extracts in HL-60 human promyelocytic leukemia cells. *J. Med. Food.* 2004; 7(1):13–8. [PubMed: 15117547]

[83] Ceesay MM, Vadher B, Tinwell B, Goderya R, Sawicka E. Spontaneous remission of T lymphoblastic lymphoma. *J. Clin. Pathol.* 2008; 61(8):955–7. [PubMed: 18663057]

Chapter 8

NEUROPROTECTIVE EFFECTS OF POMEGRANATES

ABSTRACT

Pomegranates have been used for centuries to treat and manage neurological disorders due to their polyphenolic antioxidant and anti-inflammatory components which represents an alternative to α-tocopherol. Pomegranates have been shown to ameliorate the deleterious effects of oxidative stress and amyloid pathology in transgenic mice models. The inherent constituents of pomegranates have been shown to inhibit the combined oxidative and neuroinflammatory damage. However, the precise mechanism of action of pomegranates in brain disorders is yet to be established. In this section, we will discuss the neuroprotective effects of pomegranates to reduce oxidative damage and neuroinflammation. This may pave the way for the development of improved treatment regimens containing pomegranate extracts to establish greater neuroprotection in several neurodegenerative disorders, and AD in particular.

INTRODUCTION

It is well established that inflammation and oxidative stress play a major role in β-amyloid (Aβ) aggregation, which may participate in the pathogenesis of Alzheimer's disease (AD) and other neurodegenerative disorders [1, 2]. Several epidemiological studies have shown that long-term use of nonsteroidal anti-inflammatory drugs (NSAIDs) can reduce the onset and slow down the progression of AD [3-11]. It has been demonstrated that chronic NSAID treatment can attenuate neuroinflammation in a variety of AD animal models, including the Tg2576 transgenic mouse expressing the amyloid precursor protein with a Swedish mutant (APPsw), and aged rats intraventrically infused with Aβ [11]. Despite the potential protective effects of NSAIDs for the prevention of AD, the use of these drugs is limited due to adverse effects in the gastrointestinal system, and occasional kidney and liver toxicity caused by inhibition of cyclooxygenase-I (COX-I) [12, 13]. These unwanted effects have renewed the search for alternative anti-inflammatory agents that have no effect on COX-I inhibition.

Antioxidants have also been shown to be beneficial protecting against the age-related accumulation of oxidative stress in the ageing brain, which may also be partly associated with the pathological hallmarks observed in AD [14-20]. Evidence from *in vitro* and *in vivo* studies indicating potential neuroprotective effects of antioxidants against Aβ toxicity have paved the path for clinical trials to examine the potential of pharmacological therapies to reduce free-radical damage in the brain to suppress the rate of conversion of cognitive impairment to dementia in elderly patients, and determine the beneficial effects in the ageing brain [21-27]. However, only high doses of α-tocopherol showed a marked reduction in the number of individuals developing dementia [28]. Therefore, there is a growing interest in the identification of new antioxidants, since α-tocopherol is a poor free-radical scavenger of reactive nitrogen species during the inflammatory process in AD.

Oxidative Stress and the Brain

Oxidative stress refers to the pathological state in which the production of reactive oxygen species (i.e., Free Radicals) is increased above the body's antioxidant defence capacity. Functional damage with subsequent cell death occurs as a consequence of the oxidisation of cellular components such as proteins, lipids and nuclear material (i.e., DNA). Accumulating evidence supports the role of OS in the pathogenesis of a number of neurodegenerative diseases.

The brain is particularly vulnerable to oxidative stress as it uses a large amount of oxygen and glucose for energy, generating large quantities of reactive oxygen species (ROS), and advanced glycation end products (AGE's). The brain also contains a high concentration of polyunsaturated fatty acids, which are most susceptible to oxidative damage.[3] Moreover, throughout life;

the brain is exposed to excitatory amino acids such as glutamate and other excitatory neurotransmitters that, when present in excess, induce excitotoxicity and high levels of oxidative stress.

A number of studies have demonstrated that the serum and brain tissue of patients with Alzheimer's disease (AD) is associated with increased levels of oxidative stress markers. Studies have shown that the serum of AD patients have evidence of increased DNA, protein and lipid damage.

Dementias such as AD are progressive with the eventual brain pathology thought to develop over years. Of all the possible risk factors, by far the greatest is advancing age. As neurons are the longest lived cells in the body they are also particularly vulnerable to accumulated damage. In a controlled environment, our lab has shown that Wistar rats fed a normal chow diet develop oxidative stress in the brain that accelerates markedly after middle age. Does this also occur in humans?

Other known risk factors for AD such as increased inflammation, decreased intracellular pH, elevations of brain iron levels and mitochondrial dysfunction all increase oxidative stress. Cardiovascular disease and stroke also increase the risk of developing AD and require oxidative stress in the development of their pathology. Importantly, risk factors such as high dietary fat and high cholesterol only cause disease in the presence of oxidative stress. Thus, oxidative stress seems to precede cellular and tissue damage which governs the progression of cell degenerative disease in the brain.

Psychosocial stressors and lack of physical activity have also been identified as environmental risk factors for AD. It is relevant to note that psychosocial stress increases OS and low physical activity reduces antioxidant capacity. In short, risk factors for AD also appear to be risk factors for oxidative stress. There is accumulating evidence that dietary intake of antioxidants and exercise lower oxidative damage in the periphery. Though a number of animal studies have observed changes in brain oxidative stress as a result of positive diet and lifestyle changes, no published study has yet validated this in humans. Researchers have found that individuals of Japanese and African origin living in the USA have a higher incidence of AD (4.1%, and 6.24% respectively) compared to their native soil counterparts. These findings support the theory that diet and lifestyle are important to the development of AD.

The pomegranate (Punica granatum L.) is a polyphenolic rich fruit that has been extensively referenced in medical folklore [29]. In several countries of the Arabian Peninsula and notably Yemen, pomegranates are widely used for the treatment of common ailments, including diarrhea, stomachache, healing wounds, acidosis, dysentery, microbial infections, haemorrhage and various infectious and non-infectious respiratory pathologies [30]. Phytochemicals such as polyphenols (including the phenolic acids and flavonoids which are concentrated in pomegranates) have demonstrated antioxidant properties, and can inhibit inflammation and other deleterious processes involved in degenerative diseases [31]. Pomegranate pericarp is also highly rich in tannins (gallic acid, ellagic acid), which are potent antioxidants [32]. These polyphenols have been shown to inhibit carcinogenesis [33] and display various anti-cancer properties [34]. Tannins which are present in high levels in commercially processed pomegranate juice from pressing the whole fruit and the peels, also augment the juices antioxidant power [35]. Given the polyphenols possess powerful antioxidant properties, it is likely that pomegranate juice extracts can reduce amyloid load and improve cognitive behavioral deficits in mouse models for AD, and attenuate locomotor dysfunction and neuronal pathology in PD and other neurodegenerative diseases

Clinical Applications of Pomegranates in Neurodegenerative Diseases

Pomegranates and Alzheimer's Disease

Alzheimer's disease (AD) is a progressive neurodegenerative disorder that primarily affects the elderly population. It is estimated that over 25 million individuals worldwide are affected by AD. Current statistics indicate that the number of patients suffering from AD is rising continually and represents one of the biggest challenges for most societies throughout the world (Francis et al., 1999). AD is characterized by irreversible, progressive loss of cholinergic neurons accompanied by memory deficits and dementia (Filley, 1995). At present, the aetiology of AD remains unclear. However, growing evidence has suggested that oxidative imbalance plays an important role in the pathogenesis of AD (Guidi et al., 2006). AD is the major human neurodegenerative disease and the most common cause of dementia among the elderly. Increasing evidence suggests that functional food and diet could counteract the oxidative stress associated with the disease, (Cai and Sesti, 2009; Sesti et al., 2010). Among the different types of nutrients proposed, polyphenols present in plants and fruits have shown to have beneficial anti-ageing and neuroprotective effects mediated by their antioxidant and anti-inflammatory properties (Joseph et al., 2009).

Our group showed a tendency of the pomegranate diet to improve the performance over the acquisition phase of the spatial learning, as was indicated by the residual decrease of latencies in 15-month old Tg2576 mouse. We observed improved performance of the mice fed with the pomegranate diet during the probe test at 15 months of age. That is, pomegranate-fed mice spent more time in the target quadrant and made more annulus crossings than the mice fed with the standard chow diet, which demonstrated a significant cognitive improvement. An increasing amount of studies have reported beneficial effects of other diets supplemented with different antioxidant extracts in other transgenic mouse models for AD (Joseph et al., 2003; Hartman et al., 2006).

We also found that APPsw/Tg2576 placed on a 4% pomegranate diet spent more time in the open arms of the elevated plus-maze, indicating less anxiety compared to tg mice fed standard chow. APPsw/Tg2576 control mice had significantly higher percentages of entries into the closed arms of the EPM, and spent less time in the open arms of the open field test than wild-type control mice. These behaviours were related to an anxiogenic effect induced by the deposition Aβ, and supplementation with pomegranates may reduce anxiety, which is a deleterious symptom of human AD.

Beneficial health effects of fruit and vegetables have been emphasized by several epidemiological studies. Evidence has pointed out that fruit consumption can play an important role in the prevention of age-related diseases linked to oxidative stress and neurodegeneration. Pomegranates have been revealed as a promising source of phytochemicals with a broad array of health benefits. Several studies have shown the beneficial effects of pomegranate intake in humans, and animal models of disease, including antiatherogenic, antioxidant, antihypertensive, anti-inflammatory, reduced low-density lipoprotein, and improvement of sperm quality. Pomegranate plays a role in protecting neuron cells from oxidative stress and MPTP-induced neurotoxicity. Dietary supplementation of pregnant mice with pomegranates resulted in significantly reduced brain damage to postnatal day 7 pups that were exposed to hypoxia–ischemia (Loren et al., 2005; Singh et al., 2008). Pomegranate also improved affective and motor behaviour in mice exposed to cytotoxic levels of proton radiation. Moreover, other studies have shown that pomegranates can also reduce the levels of soluble Aβ, prevent Aβ deposition and hippocampal plaque formation, and attenuate behavioural deficits in APPsw/Tg2576 mice consistent with our current findings.

It has been demonstrated that pomegranate products contain high antioxidant activity, which is directly related to their phenolic content. These biological actions have been mainly attributed to essential phenolic compounds, such as anthocyanins and ellagitannins. The high antioxidant activity of pomegranate is located mainly in the fruit's rind, due to the higher presence of punicalagins and ellagic acid derivatives. One study suggests that extracts from the pomegranate husk may contain natural inhibitors for β-secretase (BACE1), an endogenous enzyme involved in the extracellular cleavage of APP. While this study was primarily focused in examining the potential effects of pomegranate supplementation on cognitive and behavioural functions, further studies are needed to elucidate the molecular basis of these observed effects of pomegranates.

Pomegranates and Parkinson's Disease

PD represents the second most common neurological disorder after Alzheimer's disease (AD), and affects 2% of the population over the age of 60 years. PD is characterized by the chronic and progressive loss of dopaminergic neurons in the substantia nigra [36]. Although the etiology of PD is not yet known, current studies have suggested that oxidative stress may be a major player [37]. An imbalance between the formation of free radicals and reactive oxygen species (ROS), and the body's endogenous antioxidant defense mechanisms, has also been implicated in the pathogenesis of other neurodegenerative diseases such as AD, Huntington's disease (HD), Pick's disease, amyotrophic lateral sclerosis (ALS), epilepsy, schizophrenia, and hypoxic-ischemic brain injury. ROS can induce oxidative damage to lipids, nucleic acids and proteins, promote abnormal aggregation of cytoskeletal proteins, inactivate major metabolic enzymes, and facilitate mitochondrial dysfunction, and the formation of reactive nitrogen species (RNS) and advanced glycation end products formation leading to further oxidative stress formation [38-55]. Therefore, increased total antioxidant capacity has been associated with protection against neurodegeneration [47].

Although several new therapies have emerged to treat PD, these treatment strategies only provide symptomatic relief and do not affect the progression of the disease [56]. Moreover, long-term use of these drugs can induce adverse side effects which may not be tolerated by patients with PD. Therefore, newer, more effective drugs are needed that specifically target PD development. Recent studies have focused on the benefits of naturally occurring phytochemicals that exhibit potent antioxidant effects as potential neuroprotective agents [57, 58]. Pomegranate has antioxidant function that may help protect neurons against MPTP-induced neurotoxicity. The neuroprotective effects of pomegranate juice extract have been previously demonstrated using an *in vivo* transgenic animal model of AD [59]. However, the effects of pomegranate juice extract on MPTP-induced neurotoxicity in primary human neuronal cells have not been investigated previously.

The biotransformation of MPTP into MPP+, which is catalyzed by the mitochondrial enzyme monoamine oxidase B, represents the major route for MPTP-mediated neurotoxicity [60]. The conversion of MPTP to MPP^+ has been suggested to induce the formation of ROS. This notion is supported by previously studies which showed increased superoxide ($O_2^{\cdot -}$) and hydroxyl radical ($^{\cdot}OH$) levels during the biotransformation of MPTP (reviewed in [61]). While the damage induced by $O_2^{\cdot -}$ is limited, it can react with nitric oxide (NO) to form peroxynitrite ($ONOOO^-$) which readily forms the more reactive $^{\cdot}OH$ radical. Other studies have shown that MPTP induces toxicity through ATP depletion and mitochondrial dysfunction. Moreover, Kutty et al. (1991) showed that ATP depletion plays a major role in MPTP-induced neuronal cell death [62].

Our group previously showed that selected pomegranate juice extract can protect against MPTP-induced neurotoxicity in primary human neurons in a dose dependent manner by attenuating MPTP-induced increase in extracellular lactate dehydrogenase (LDH) activity, which represents a well-established measure for cell death. However, we did not observe a significant increase in lipid peroxidation, an established measure for oxidative stress. MDA is widely used to assess lipid peroxidation both *in vitro* and *in vivo* [63]. However, it is likely that MDA can form complexes with other biological components such as protein, lipids and nucleic acids which can contribute to an underestimation of endogenous lipid peroxidation [64]. On the contrary to our lipid peroxidation data, we also showed that MPTP can lead to distinct alterations in endogenous antioxidant defense mechanisms. MPTP treatment has been previously shown to significantly increased Mn-SOD and CuZn-SOD activities in the striatum of C57BL/6 mice, which is suggestive of acute oxidative stress insult [65]. SOD is up-regulated in cells when $O_2^{\cdot -}$ is produced in excessive levels [66]. This observation suggests that SOD may play a role in the toxicity observed following acute treatment of MPTP, although ROS formation may not play a major role in MPTP-induced toxicity. We also observed a significant increase in CAT after 24 hour treatment with MPTP. CAT is an enzyme that is involved in the detoxification of ROS and the elimination of hydrogen peroxide (H_2O_2) in particular [67]. The increase in both intracellular SOD and CAT activity may therefore represent an adaptive response due to the leakage of free radicals during impaired mitochondrial respiration.

Treatment with MPTP also lead to reduced activity of GPx, and decreased levels of the essential pyridine nucleotide NAD+, and ATP and GSH in primary human neurons after 24 hour exposure. The maintenance of GPx activity appears crucial for the maintenance of cell viability during oxidative insult [68-71]. One study showed that increased GPx expression could protect against H_2O_2-mediated oxidative stress due to methamphetamine as measured by extracellular LDH activity [72]. Moreover, previous studies have shown that MPP+, the metabolite of MPTP induces GSH depletion without increasing the levels of oxidized glutathione disulfide (GSSG) [73]. Reduced GSH levels may occur due to MPP+ induced decline in intracellular NAD+ and ATP stores which are necessary for GSH anabolism, release and consequent hydrolysis. Taken together, our data suggests that MPTP exposure can limit the endogenous antioxidant defense, subsequently increasing the vulnerability of neuronal cells to additional oxidative stress. An imbalance in the function of endogenous antioxidant defense mechanisms can lead to the accumulation of free radicals and ROS and increased susceptibility to oxidative stress, which contributes to the pathogenesis of PD.

Different brain cell types are used to study the effects of oxidative stress in culture.

Although our data relate to foetal neuronal cultures, it is likely that our results also reflect what is happening in adult astrocytes and neurons. Human cell culture models have demonstrated a neuroprotective role of both astrocytes and microglial cells against ROS mediated neuronal cell death. However, at the same time, evidence exist linking neurotoxicity to oxidative-stress mediated astrocyte/microglial activation [74, 75]. We have previously shown that the inflammatory profile is conserved between human and simian adult and foetal astrocytes and neurons [76, 77]. Therefore, human foetal brain cells are a relevant model to study neurodegenerative diseases and MPTP-induced toxicity in particular.

Pomegranate juice extract is known to exhibit anti-oxidant and anti-inflammatory properties. pomegranate juice extract has been shown to have a variety of protective effects in several disease models, including reduced low-density lipoprotein (LDL) aggregation, oxidative stress, amyloid load and improved cognitive behaviour in AD mice [78-86]. Nevertheless, the effect of pomegranate juice extract against the MPTP toxicity in human neurons has not been previously investigated. Our data shows that pomegranate juice extract can reverse the effect of MPTP on the activities of antioxidant enzymes and attenuate MPTP induced toxicity in a dose dependent manner. An assessment of total phenolic compounds suggests that the neuroprotective effects of polyphenols are dependent on their total phenolic concentration [87-90].

Our findings show that pomegranate juice extract at the stated concentrations has no toxic effect on human neurons and may therefore be therapeutically safe. However, little information is available in the literature regarding the absorption, bioavailability, biodistribution, and metabolism of important bioactive constituents found in pomegranate juice extract, such as phenolic acids, flavonoids, and tannins [91]. An *in vitro* study of the digestion of pomegranate phenolic compounds showed that these molecules are present during digestion in relatively large amounts (29%). However, anthocyanins are metabolised or degraded (97%). Seeram et al. (2008) investigated the bioavailability of polyphenols derived from pomegranate juice extract in liquid and lypophilised form. Plasma bioavailability, determined by examining GAE levels 6 hours after consumption, was not statistically different between the 2 interventions. The time of maximum concentration was delayed in the polyphenol powder extract (2.58 ± 0.42 h) compared with pomegranate juice (0.65 ± 0.23 h) and polyphenol liquid extract (0.94 ± 0.06 h) [92]. It is likely that the bioavailability of pomegranate polyphenols may be affected by several factors, including individual variability, differential processing of pomegranate juice, and the analytical techniques employed to detect low postprandial concentrations of these metabolites [93]. In conclusion, pomegranate juice extract provide protection against the neurotoxic effects of MPTP in human neurons, and the mechanisms of protection may be related to their antioxidant activity and botanical phenolic constituents. The potential neuroprotective effects of pomegranate juice extract warrant further investigation.

Neonatal Hypoxic-Ischemic Brain Injury

Neonatal hypoxic-ischemic (HI) brain injury in severely preterm, very low birth-weight infants is a major cause of infant illness and death. This effect has been partly attributed to an increase in the production of reactive oxygen species. Supplementation of pomegranate juice in drinking water has been shown to significantly reduce brain tissue loss (64% decrease) and significantly decreased hippocampal caspase-3 activity (84% decrease) compared to mouse neonates with experimentally-induced HI brain injury from dams who consumed a control beverage.

FUTURE PROSPECTS AND CONCLUSION

During the last few years, antioxidants have received special attention as dietary supplements for the prevention and treatment of AD. Many studies have suggested that reversals in age-related memory declines might be accomplished by increasing the dietary intake rich in antioxidant activity. Recently, numerous lines of evidence have demonstrated that non-nutritive bioactive chemicals found in plants can improve cognitive function and inhibit the formation and extension of Aβ fibrils and reduce plaque burden. Fruits are a good source of vital bioactive compounds. Pomegranates (*Punica granatum Linn.*) contain very high levels of polyphenols as compared to other fruits and vegetables. Pomegranates have been extensively used in Unani, Ayurvedic and Chinese systems of medicine due to their high polyphenolic properties. There are a number of commercially available polyphenol-rich pomegranate beverages, which base their marketing strategies on antioxidant potency and are likely to play a neuroprotective role in the treatment of neurodegenerative diseases in the near future.

REFERENCES

[1] Mattson, M.P., Oxidative stress, perturbed calcium homeostasis, and immune dysfunction in Alzheimer's disease. *J Neurovirol*, 2002. 8(6): p. 539-50.

[2] Mattson, M.P., Pathway towards and away from Azheimer's Disease. *Nature*, 2004. 430: p. 630-639.

[3] Blom, M.A., et al., NSAIDS inhibit the IL-1 beta-induced IL-6 release from human post-mortem astrocytes: the involvement of prostaglandin E2. *Brain Res,* 1997. 777(1-2): p. 210-8.

[4] Dairam, A., P. Chetty, and S. Daya, Non-steroidal anti-inflammatory agents, tolmetin and sulindac, attenuate oxidative stress in rat brain homogenate and reduce quinolinic acid-induced neurodegeneration in rat hippocampal neurons. *Metab Brain Dis*, 2006.

[5] Doraiswamy, P.M., Non-cholinergic strategies for treating and preventing Alzheimer's disease. *CNS Drugs*, 2002. 16(12): p. 811-24.

[6] Eriksen, J.L., et al., NSAIDs and enantiomers of flurbiprofen target gamma-secretase and lower Abeta 42 in vivo. *J Clin Invest,* 2003. 112(3): p. 440-9.

[7] Ferencik, M., et al., Alzheimer's disease, inflammation and non-steroidal anti-inflammatory drugs. *Bratisl Lek Listy*, 2001. 102(3): p. 123-32.

[8] Gottlieb, S., NSAIDs can lower risk of Alzheimer's. *BMJ*, 2001. 323: p. 1269.

[9] Hull, M., K. Lieb, and B.L. Fiebich, Pathways of inflammatory activation in Alzheimer's disease: potential targets for disease modifying drugs. *Curr Med Chem*, 2002. 9(1): p. 83-8.

[10] Lim, G.P., et al., Ibuprofen suppresses plaque pathology and inflammation in a mouse model for Alzheimer's disease. *J Neurosci,* 2000. 20(15): p. 5709-14.

[11] Morihara, T., et al., Ibuprofen suppresses interleukin-1beta induction of pro-amyloidogenic alpha1-antichymotrypsin to ameliorate beta-amyloid (Abeta) pathology in Alzheimer's models. *Neuropsychopharmacology*, 2005. 30(6): p. 1111-20.

[12] Szekely, C.A., et al., Nonsteroidal anti-inflammatory drugs for the prevention of Alzheimer's disease: a systematic review. *Neuroepidemiology*, 2004. 23(4): p. 159-69.

[13] Zandi, P.P. and J.C. Breitner, Do NSAIDs prevent Alzheimer's disease? And, if so, why? The epidemiological evidence. *Neurobiol Aging,* 2001. 22(6): p. 811-7.

[14] Schmitt, B., et al., Combination therapy in Alzheimer's disease: a review of current evidence. *CNS Drugs*, 2004. 18(13): p. 827-44.

[15] Smith, J.V. and Y. Luo, Elevation of oxidative free radicals in Alzheimer's disease models can be attenuated by Ginkgo biloba extract EGb 761. *J Alzheimers Dis*, 2003. 5(4): p. 287-300.

[16] Tariot, P.N. and H.J. Federoff, Current treatment for Alzheimer disease and future prospects. *Alzheimer Dis Assoc Disord*, 2003. 17 Suppl 4: p. S105-13.

[17] Varadarajan, S., et al., Review: Alzheimer's amyloid beta-peptide-associated free radical oxidative stress and neurotoxicity. *J Struct Biol,* 2000. 130(2-3): p. 184-208.

[18] Zandi, P.P., et al., Reduced risk of Alzheimer disease in users of antioxidant vitamin supplements: the Cache County Study. *Arch Neurol,* 2004. 61(1): p. 82-8.

[19] Zandi, P.P., J.C. Breitner, and J.C. Anthony, Is pharmacological prevention of Alzheimer's a realistic goal? *Expert Opin Pharmacother,* 2002. 3(4): p. 365-80.
[20] Zbarsky, V., et al., Neuroprotective properties of natural phenolic antioxidants curcumin and naringenin but not quercetin and fisetin in a 6-OHDA model of Parkinson's disease. *Free Radic Res,* 2005. 39: p. 1119-1125.
[21] Doraiswamy, P.M. and G.L. Xiong, Pharmacological strategies for the prevention of Alzheimer's disease. *Expert Opin Pharmacother*, 2006. 7(1): p. 1-10.
[22] Floyd, R.A., Antioxidants, oxidative stress, and degenerative neurological disorders. *Proc Soc Exp Biol Med*, 1999. 222(3): p. 236-45.
[23] Frank, B. and S. Gupta, A review of antioxidants and Alzheimer's disease. *Ann Clin Psychiatry*, 2005. 17(4): p. 269-86.
[24] Halliwell, B., Role of free radicals in the neurodegenerative diseases: therapeutic implications for antioxidant treatment. *Drugs Aging*, 2001. 18(9): p. 685-716.
[25] Lehtinen, M.K. and A. Bonni, Modeling oxidative stress in the central nervous system. *Curr Mol Med,* 2006. 6(8): p. 871-81.
[26] Michaelis, M.L., Drugs targeting Alzheimer's disease: some things old and some things new. *J Pharmacol Exp Ther*, 2003. 304(3): p. 897-904.
[27] Rao, A.V. and B. Balachandran, Role of oxidative stress and antioxidants in neurodegenerative diseases. *Nutr Neurosci*, 2002. 5(5): p. 291-309.
[28] Smith, C.D., et al., Excess brain protein oxidation and enzyme dysfunction in normal aging and in Alzheimer disease. P*roc Natl Acad Sci U S A*, 1991. 88(23): p. 10540-3.
[29] Langley, P., Why a pomegranate? *BMJ*, 2000. 321(7269): p. 1153-4.
[30] Vidal, A., et al., Studies on the toxicity of Punica granatum L. (Punicaceae) whole fruit extracts. *J Ethnopharmacol,* 2003. 89(2-3): p. 295-300.
[31] Aggarwal, B.B. and S. Shishodia, Suppression of the nuclear factor-kappaB activation pathway by spice-derived phytochemicals: reasoning for seasoning. *Ann N Y Acad Sci,* 2004. 1030: p. 434-41.
[32] Ashoori, F., et al., Involvement of lipid peroxidation in necrosis of skin flaps and its suppression by ellagic acid. *Plast Reconstr Surg*, 1994. 94(7): p. 1027-37.
[33] Hirose, M., et al., Inhibitory effects of 1-O-hexyl-2,3,5-trimethylhydroquinone (HTHQ), green tea catechins and other

antioxidants on 2-amino-6-methyldipyrido[1,2-a:3',2'-d]imidazole (Glu-P-1)-induced rat hepatocarcinogenesis and dose-dependent inhibition by HTHQ of lesion induction by Glu-P-1 or 2-amino-3,8-dimethylimidazo[4,5-f]quinoxaline (MeIQx). *Carcinogenesis*, 1995. 16(12): p. 3049-55.

[34] Kim, N.D., et al., Chemopreventive and adjuvant therapeutic potential of pomegranate (Punica granatum) for human breast cancer. *Breast Cancer Res Treat*, 2002. 71(3): p. 203-17.

[35] Gil, M.I., et al., Antioxidant activity of pomegranate juice and its relationship with phenolic composition and processing. *J Agric Food Chem*, 2000. 48(10): p. 4581-9.

[36] Lo Bianco, C., et al., Lentiviral vector delivery of parkin prevents dopaminergic degeneration in an alpha-synuclein rat model of Parkinson's disease. *Proc Natl Acad Sci U S A*, 2004. 101(50): p. 17510-5.

[37] Mandel, S., et al., Neuroprotective strategies in Parkinson's disease : an update on progress. *CNS Drugs*, 2003. 17(10): p. 729-62.

[38] Butterfield, P.G., Environment: seeking clues to Parkinson's disease. *Reflections*, 1996. 22(3): p. 14-5.

[39] Markesbery, W.R., Neuropathological criteria for the diagnosis of Alzheimer's disease. *Neurobiol Aging*, 1997. 18(4 Suppl): p. S13-9.

[40] Ball, M.J. and G.H. Murdoch, Neuropathological criteria for the diagnosis of Alzheimer's disease: are we really ready yet? *Neurobiol Aging*, 1997. 18(4 Suppl): p. S3-12.

[41] Kumar, H., et al., Nuclear factor erythroid 2 - related factor 2 signaling in Parkinson disease: a promising multi therapeutic target against oxidative stress, neuroinflammation and cell death. *CNS Neurol Disord Drug Targets*, 2012. 11(8): p. 1015-29.

[42] Yan, M.H., X. Wang, and X. Zhu, Mitochondrial defects and oxidative stress in Alzheimer disease and Parkinson disease. *Free Radic Biol Med,* 2012.

[43] Perfeito, R., T. Cunha-Oliveira, and A.C. Rego, Revisiting oxidative stress and mitochondrial dysfunction in the pathogenesis of Parkinson disease--resemblance to the effect of amphetamine drugs of abuse. *Free Radic Biol Med,* 2012. 53(9): p. 1791-806.

[44] Jeong, H.J., et al., Transduced Tat-DJ-1 protein protects against oxidative stress-induced SH-SY5Y cell death and Parkinson disease in a mouse model. *Mol Cells,* 2012. 33(5): p. 471-8.

[45] Chien, W.L., et al., Impairment of oxidative stress-induced heme oxygenase-1 expression by the defect of Parkinson-related gene of PINK1. *J Neurochem*, 2011. 117(4): p. 643-53.
[46] Bayir, H., et al., Peroxidase mechanism of lipid-dependent cross-linking of synuclein with cytochrome C: protection against apoptosis versus delayed oxidative stress in Parkinson disease. *J Biol Chem*, 2009. 284(23): p. 15951-69.
[47] Henchcliffe, C. and M.F. Beal, Mitochondrial biology and oxidative stress in Parkinson disease pathogenesis. *Nat Clin Pract Neurol*, 2008. 4(11): p. 600-9.
[48] Bloomer, R.J., et al., Effect of resistance training on blood oxidative stress in Parkinson disease. *Med Sci Sports Exerc*, 2008. 40(8): p. 1385-9.
[49] Nunomura, A., et al., Neuronal death and survival under oxidative stress in Alzheimer and Parkinson diseases. *CNS Neurol Disord Drug Targets*, 2007. 6(6): p. 411-23.
[50] Battisti, C., et al., Oxidative-stress-induced apoptosis in PBLs of two patients with Parkinson disease secondary to alpha-synuclein mutation. *J Neurol Sci*, 2008. 267(1-2): p. 120-4.
[51] Yamamoto, N., et al., Proteasome inhibition induces glutathione synthesis and protects cells from oxidative stress: relevance to Parkinson disease. *J Biol Chem*, 2007. 282(7): p. 4364-72.
[52] Ebadi, M. and S. Sharma, Metallothioneins 1 and 2 attenuate peroxynitrite-induced oxidative stress in Parkinson disease. *Exp Biol Med (Maywood),* 2006. 231(9): p. 1576-83.
[53] Veech, G.A., et al., Disrupted mitochondrial electron transport function increases expression of anti-apoptotic bcl-2 and bcl-X(L) proteins in SH-SY5Y neuroblastoma and in Parkinson disease cybrid cells through oxidative stress. *J Neurosci Res*, 2000. 61(6): p. 693-700.
[54] Gonzalez-Fraguela, M.E., et al. [Indicators of oxidative stress and the effect of antioxidant treatment in patients with primary Parkinson disease]. *Rev Neurol*, 1998. 26(149): p. 28-33.
[55] Castellani, R., et al., Glycoxidation and oxidative stress in Parkinson disease and diffuse Lewy body disease. *Brain Res,* 1996. 737(1-2): p. 195-200.
[56] Cordesse, V., et al. [Analysis of clinical pathway in changing and disabling neurological diseases.]. *Rev Neurol (Paris)*, 2013.

[57] Houghton, P.J. and M.J. Howes, Natural products and derivatives affecting neurotransmission relevant to Alzheimer's and Parkinson's disease. *Neurosignals*, 2005. 14(1-2): p. 6-22.

[58] Mythri, R.B., G. Harish, and M.M. Bharath, Therapeutic potential of natural products in Parkinson's disease. *Recent Pat Endocr Metab Immune Drug Discov,* 2012. 6(3): p. 181-200.

[59] Hartman, R.E., et al., Pomegranate juice decreases amyloid load and improves behavior in a mouse model of Alzheimer's disease. *Neurobiol Dis*, 2006. 24(3): p. 506-15.

[60] Markey, S.P., et al., Intraneuronal generation of a pyridinium metabolite may cause drug-induced parkinsonism. *Nature*, 1984. 311(5985): p. 464-7.

[61] Ho, P.W., et al., Mitochondrial neuronal uncoupling proteins: a target for potential disease-modification in Parkinson's disease. *Transl Neurodegener*, 2012. 1(1): p. 3.

[62] Kutty, R.K., et al., MPTP-induced ATP depletion and cell death in neuroblastoma X glioma hybrid NG 108-15 cells: protection by glucose and sensitization by tetraphenylborate. *Toxicol Appl Pharmacol,* 1991. 107(2): p. 377-88.

[63] Dalle-Donne, I., et al., Biomarkers of oxidative damage in human disease. *Clin Chem*, 2006. 52(4): p. 601-23.

[64] Shulaev, V. and D.J. Oliver, Metabolic and proteomic markers for oxidative stress. New tools for reactive oxygen species research. *Plant Physiol,* 2006. 141(2): p. 367-72.

[65] Thiffault, C., et al., Effect of MPTP and L-deprenyl on antioxidant enzymes and lipid peroxidation levels in mouse brain. *J Neurochem,* 1995. 65(6): p. 2725-33.

[66] Kar, S. and M. Kavdia, Endothelial NO and O Production Rates Differentially Regulate Oxidative, Nitroxidative and Nitrosative Stress in the Microcirculation. *Free Radic Biol Med*, 2013.

[67] Ribeiro, L.C., et al., Caloric restriction improves basal redox parameters in hippocampus and cerebral cortex of Wistar rats. *Brain Res*, 2012. 1472: p. 11-9.

[68] Dokic, I., et al., Glutathione peroxidase 1 activity dictates the sensitivity of glioblastoma cells to oxidative stress. *Glia*, 2012. 60(11): p. 1785-800.

[69] Esposito, L.A., et al., Mitochondrial oxidative stress in mice lacking the glutathione peroxidase-1 gene. *Free Radic Biol Med*, 2000. 28(5): p. 754-66.

[70] Inoue, Y., et al., Oxidative stress response in yeast: glutathione peroxidase of Hansenula mrakii is bound to the membrane of both mitochondria and cytoplasm. *Biochim Biophys Acta*, 1995. 1245(3): p. 325-30.

[71] Doroshow, J.H., Glutathione peroxidase and oxidative stress. *Toxicol Lett*, 1995. 82-83: p. 395-8.

[72] Hom, D.G., et al., Elevated expression of glutathione peroxidase in PC12 cells results in protection against methamphetamine but not MPTP toxicity. *Brain Res Mol Brain Res*, 1997. 46(1-2): p. 154-60.

[73] Drechsel, D.A., L.P. Liang, and M. Patel, 1-methyl-4-phenylpyridinium-induced alterations of glutathione status in immortalized rat dopaminergic neurons. *Toxicol Appl Pharmacol*, 2007. 220(3): p. 341-8.

[74] Hirrlinger, J., et al., Microglial cells in culture express a prominent glutathione system for the defense against reactive oxygen species. *Developmental Neuroscience*, 2000. 22(5-6): p. 384-392.

[75] Hirrlinger, J., B. Hamprecht, and R. Dringen, Application and modulation of a permanent hydrogen peroxide-induced oxidative stress to cultured astroglial cells. *Brain Research Protocols*, 1999. 4(2): p. 223-229.

[76] Croitoru-Lamoury, J., et al., Expression of chemokines and their receptors in human and simian astrocytes: Evidence for a central role of TNF alpha and IFN gamma in CXCR4 and CCR5 modulation. *Glia*, 2003. 41(4): p. 354-370.

[77] Guillemin, G.J., et al., Quinolinic acid upregulates chemokine production and chemokine receptor expression in astrocytes. *Glia*, 2003. 41(4): p. 371-81.

[78] Aviram, M., Pomegranate juice as a major source for polyphenolic flavonoids and it is most potent antioxidant against LDL oxidation and atherosclerosis. *Xi Biennial Meeting of the Society for Free Radical Research International*, 2002: p. 523-528.

[79] Aviram, M., Pomegranate juice as a major source for polyphenolic flavonoids and it is most potent antioxidant against LDL oxidation and atherosclerosis. *Free Radical Biology and Medicine*, 2002. 33: p. S139-S140.

[80] Aviram, M., et al., Pomegranate juice consumption for 3 years by patients with carotid artery stenosis reduces common carotid intima-media thickness, blood pressure and LDL oxidation (vol 23, pg 423, 2004). *Clinical Nutrition*, 2008. 27(4): p. 671-671.

[81] Bandeira Sde, M., et al., Characterization of Blood Oxidative Stress in Type 2 Diabetes Mellitus Patients: Increase in Lipid Peroxidation and SOD Activity. *Oxid Med Cell Longev*, 2012. 2012: p. 819310.

[82] Butterfield, A., A.M. Swomley, and R. Sultana, Amyloid beta-Peptide 1-42-induced Oxidative Stress in Alzheimer Disease: Importance in Disease Pathogenesis and Progression. *Antioxid Redox Signal*, 2012.

[83] Mori-Okamoto, J., et al., Pomegranate extract improves a depressive state and bone properties in menopausal syndrome model ovariectomized mice. *Journal of Ethnopharmacology*, 2004. 92(1): p. 93-101.

[84] Rosenblat, M. and M. Aviram, Antioxidants as Targeted Therapy: A Special Protective Role for Pomegranate and Paraoxonases (PONs). *Asymptomatic Atherosclerosis: Pathophysiology, Detection and Treatment*, 2010: p. 621-634.

[85] Rosenblat, M., T. Hayek, and M. Aviram, Anti-oxidative effects of pomegranate juice (PJ) consumption by diabetic patients on serum and on macrophages. *Atherosclerosis*, 2006. 187(2): p. 363-371.

[86] Rosenblat, M., N. Volkova, and M. Aviram, Pomegranate juice (PJ) consumption antioxidative properties on mouse macrophages, but not PJ beneficial effects on macrophage cholesterol and triglyceride metabolism, are mediated via PJ-induced stimulation of macrophage PON2. *Atherosclerosis*, 2010. 212(1): p. 86-92.

[87] Panickar, K.S. and S. Jang, Dietary and Plant Polyphenols Exert Neuroprotective Effects and Improve Cognitive Function in Cerebral Ischemia. *Recent Pat Food Nutr Agric*, 2013.

[88] Panickar, K.S., Bioactive components of plant products including polyphenols exert neuroprotective effects and benefit neural function. *Cent Nerv Syst Agents Med Chem*, 2013. 13(1): p. 2.

[89] Tavares, L., et al., Neuroprotective effects of digested polyphenols from wild blackberry species. *Eur J Nutr*, 2013. 52(1): p. 225-36.

[90] Essa, M.M., et al., Neuroprotective effect of natural products against Alzheimer's disease. *Neurochem Res*, 2012. 37(9): p. 1829-42.

[91] Petti, S. and C. Scully, Polyphenols, oral health and disease: A review. *Journal of Dentistry*, 2009. 37(6): p. 413-423.

[92] Seeram, N.P., et al., Pomegranate juice and extracts provide similar levels of plasma and urinary ellagitannin metabolites in human subjects. J*ournal of Medicinal Food*, 2008. 11(2): p. 390-394.

[93] Basu, A. and K. Penugonda, Pomegranate juice: a heart-healthy fruit juice. *Nutrition Reviews*, 2009. 67(1): p. 49-56.

INDEX

B

C

F

G

H

I

J

K

L

M

P

T

U

V

W

X

Y